SECOND EDITION

HEALTH LITERACY
FROM A TO Z

Practical Ways to Communicate Your Health Message

Helen Osborne, MEd, OTR/L
President, Health Literacy Consulting
Natick, MA

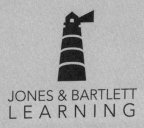

JONES & BARTLETT
LEARNING

World Headquarters
Jones & Bartlett Learning
5 Wall Street
Burlington, MA 01803
978-443-5000
info@jblearning.com
www.jblearning.com

Jones & Bartlett Learning books and products are available through most bookstores and online booksellers. To contact Jones & Bartlett Learning directly, call 800-832-0034, fax 978-443-8000, or visit our website, www.jblearning.com.

Substantial discounts on bulk quantities of Jones & Bartlett Learning publications are available to corporations, professional associations, and other qualified organizations. For details and specific discount information, contact the special sales department at Jones & Bartlett Learning via the above contact information or send an email to specialsales@jblearning.com.

Production Credits
Publisher: David D. Cella
Managing Editor: Maro Gartside
Editorial Assistant: Teresa Reilly
Senior Production Editor: Renée Sekerak
Production Assistant: Sean Coombs
Marketing Manager: Grace Richards
Manufacturing and Inventory Control Supervisor: Amy Bacus
Composition: Cenveo Publisher Services
Cover Design: Kristin E. Parker
Cover Image: © lenetstan/ShutterStock, Inc.
Printing and Binding: Malloy, Inc.
Cover Printing: Malloy, Inc.

About the Author photo: Courtesy of Jane Hammond-Clarke

Library of Congress Cataloging-in-Publication Data

Osborne, Helen, 1948-
  Health literacy from A to Z : practical ways to communicate your health message/Helen Osborne. —2nd ed.
     p. ; cm.
  Includes bibliographical references and index.
  ISBN 978-1-4496-0053-2 (pbk.)
  I. Title.
  [DNLM: 1. Health Literacy. 2. Communication. WA 590]
  LC-classification not assigned
    613'.071—dc23   2011031271

6048
Printed in the United States of America
15 14 13 12 11   10 9 8 7 6 5 4 3 2 1

This book is dedicated to health literacy advocates everywhere. Together, we truly make it easier for others to understand and act on health information.

Contents

Foreword

For the past 45 years, I've been able to work in health care as a clerk, manager, administrator, executive, teacher, and student. Exceptional circumstances at three Massachusetts healthcare organizations—the Children's Hospital in Boston, the Dana-Farber Cancer Institute (DFCI) in Boston, and the Institute for Healthcare Improvement (IHI) in Cambridge—allowed me to gain early experience and be part of the leading edge of patient- and family-centered care (PFCC). Along the way I discovered the power and privilege of PFCC as care that is anchored in four concepts: dignity and respect, information sharing, participation, and collaboration at every level of care. In pursuit of achieving PFCC for those patients and families whom I served, I met and ultimately partnered with Helen Osborne.

We first met about 15 years ago when Helen was presenting on health literacy at DFCI. Dana-Farber was examining gaps in its practice and discovering the enormous power of the patient and family in care. We needed to learn how to move beyond aspiration to action and engagement; Helen was a teacher and guide. In the years since, Helen and I have worked together on other projects and initiatives, including simplifying IHI materials for the public and expanding personal and public engagement as part of the important Massachusetts health reform journey.

Much has changed in PFCC in recent years. Today, whether you look at the strategic plan for the U.S. Department of Health and Human Services or a strategic plan for a small rural healthcare organization, you will see an exceptional push and priority placed on PFCC and on personal and public engagement in health and health care. Surveys demonstrate that over 90 percent of healthcare organizations have been optimizing the patient experience as one of their top five strategic priorities, and 35 percent have set it as their top priority. Essential to achieving this goal, and the goals of PFCC, is meeting patients where they are, at their current knowledge base. A cornerstone of achieving this is ensuring effective communication and health literacy.

During a recent tour of a children's hospital, I asked a literacy expert what delighted her in her work. She told me the story of a boy hospitalized with a very serious cancer. He was receiving many medications, and his healthcare team was preparing to transition him to home. His mother was bilingual but unable to read or write in either language. Staff asked how she could possibly take care of her son if she couldn't read the bottle labels. It was obvious to the staff that she was a very caring mother. One staff member, working with the mother and a pharmacist, came up with a color-coded system for all the medications, which enabled the mother to administer them perfectly in the home. The mother and the staff member were thrilled.

Healthcare delivery revolves around a seemingly endless process of communicating health information clearly and ensuring it is understood correctly. It is hard for those of us (patients, family members, clinicians, colleagues, and leaders) doing the communicating. We are all in very different places. It is also hard for those of us doing the listening. We're coming from many different cultures and literacy levels, and we are scared, busy, confused, and a lot more. Patients and family members have told me for 40 years that I ask them all what they think but then don't stop talking long enough to listen. Telling healthcare professionals just to work harder and to do it better won't get us to where we need to be. Making it up as we go along won't get us what we want.

In recent years I've had some relevant profound learning as a leader. Our systems are too complex to expect ordinary people to perform perfectly 100 percent of the time. We, as leaders, must put in place systems (structures, processes, tools, and techniques) to support safe and effective practice. These systems include communications and specifically all that health literacy has to offer. Helen's efforts make up an exceptional gift in this space.

Reading Helen's whole book (all 42 chapters) honestly wasn't my original plan prior to writing the foreword, but in the end I did. As I started skimming, I realized that I was learning a lot and went back to the beginning. I also realized that this book would help me not only in my interactions in care, but also in leadership, in teaching, in my community, and in my home. It wasn't a "read" but a reference, and a just-in-time resource from which I could seek counsel—for example, just before meeting with someone who is scared, deaf, or emotional. The chapter on document design is helpful for anyone who writes, and the ever-present "Stories from Practice" ground the content in real-life experience. The almost encyclopedic "Sources to Learn More" feature in every chapter is a wonderful alternative to the Google search with a million hits. Content from the chapter on storytelling will no doubt find its way into my Harvard School of Public Health course on leading change.

As a healthcare professional I am proud to be writing this foreword. I know through experience (the name we give to our mistakes) that we will achieve exceptional and reliable results in health and health care when we engage and build the system around the patients, their families, and the public we are privileged to serve. Full engagement will require dramatic improvements in communication, listening, and understanding, and it will build on a strong foundation of systems, processes, tools, and techniques. Few things are more important in the remarkably diverse world we live in than health literacy. Helen's book is an exceptional read, tool, reference, encyclopedia, and just-in-time guide for staff at the front line, healthcare executives, and policy analysts.

This foreword began by noting the four concepts that make up patient- and family-centered care. I would like to end it on the first one, dignity and respect. Above and beyond everything else, *Health Literacy from A to Z: Practical Ways to Communicate Your Health Message, Second Edition* is anchored in the core value of respect. To me, nothing could be more important or worthwhile. I thank Helen and all involved for their effort and recommend this book to all.

Jim Conway
Adjunct Faculty, Harvard School of Public Health
Senior Fellow, Institute for Healthcare Improvement

How to Use This Book

The *Second Edition* of *Health Literacy from A to Z: Practical Ways to Communicate Your Health Message*, is written for someone who cares a lot about communicating health messages clearly and simply. It is also written for someone to whom health literacy is just one of many projects competing for time and attention. In other words, this book is written for you.

Regardless of your profession or practice setting, you probably are wearing one or more health literacy "hats." I categorize these as: (1) Producers—who are responsible for day-to-day health communication be it in print, in person, or on the Web; (2) Polishers—who manage, edit, or otherwise influence someone else's written, oral, or other communication; and (3) Policy makers—who establish policies, set standards, and work to ensure that these are met. Regardless of which health literacy hat or hats you wear, this book is designed to help.

What is health literacy? Health literacy is about communicating health information in ways that others can understand. It has three central components: communication skills of the person expressing a message; learning needs of each person receiving the message; complexity of the message itself. Each can vary for infinite reasons. That's why it is so hard to communicate health messages simply. Nonetheless, it is vital that we do.

How does this book help? This book is intended as an easy-to-use guide to be used as a starting place for your health communications. It is written in a way to inform and inspire you, not overwhelm you.

There are 42 stand-alone chapters. You can read as much or as little as you need to know now. Later, you can always read more. The chapters are arranged alphabetically from A to Z, and each includes:

- **Starting Points.** Introductory information providing context for the strategies that follow.
- **Strategies, Ideas, and Suggestions.** Lots and lots of practical, how-to ways of communicating health messages clearly and simply.
- **Stories from Practice.** Real-life experiences from a wide range of perspectives. These help make key points "come alive."

- **Citations.** References used within each chapter. These include many of my articles, podcasts, and interviews with health literacy leaders, champions, and researchers.
- **Sources to Learn More.** Extensive listing of books, articles, Web sites, podcasts, and additional resources to continue learning about each topic.

Admittedly, it was challenging for me to find the just-right words and examples—especially when writing for an audience from diverse backgrounds, interests, and levels of experience. As needed, please substitute your words and examples for mine. For instance:

- When I use the term "providers," you might instead think of doctors, nurses, technicians, therapists, pharmacists, health educators, practice managers, public health specialists, writers, graphic designers, librarians, agency directors, or teachers.
- Instead of "patients," it might be more meaningful for you to think of families, caregivers, the general public, patrons, members, Web site visitors, or students.
- When an example takes place in the clinic, feel free to think of a similar situation happening in your community center, classroom, library, or other practice setting.

For better or worse, the field of health literacy has been around long enough to develop its own jargon. Here are some terms I often use that you might not already know:

- "Intended audience." I use this as an overall term to refer to those we are trying to reach with health messages. Your audience may be one person, or many. Your audience can be local, from across the country, or from around the world.
- "Teach-back" and "feedback." These are methods to confirm understanding. Teach-back is generally used when communicating verbally. Feedback is the process of testing materials with those representing your intended audience.
- Health literacy "ally," "champion," or "advocate." These refer to you—someone who is convinced that health literacy matters, knows that health communication can and should be improved, and is determined to make a long-lasting difference.

***What's new in the* Second Edition?** When I agreed to write this *Second Edition*, I heard from other authors that doing so is often harder than writing a book the first time. Now I know that's true. But I also discovered that the process of updating, reorganizing, and rewriting is exceptionally exciting and energizing. Here are some highlights of what's new in the *Second Edition* of *Health Literacy from A to Z: Practical Ways to Communicate Your Health Message.*

New health literacy topics include: Business Side of Health Literacy; Communicating When Patients Feel Scared, Sick, and Overwhelmed; General Public: Talking with Patients About What They Learn from the Media; Organizational Efforts: Health Literacy at the Community, State, and National Levels; Regulatory and Legal Language; and Writing for the Web.

Also new in the *Second Edition*:

- Expanded focus on knowing your audience. Seven chapters offer in-depth information about: (1) children and youth, (2) culture and language, (3) emotions and cognition, (4) hearing loss, (5) literacy, (6) older adults, and (7) vision problems.
- Timely information about technology: (1) audio podcasts, (2) blogs and social media, (3) email and text messages, and (4) interactive multimedia.
- "Stories from Practice," one or more stories in each chapter that highlight real-life solutions to everyday problems.
- Checklists. Intended to remind and encourage you to put health literacy strategies into action. These three checklists are tools you can use in practice, when teaching, and with patients.

How to keep learning about health literacy? The field of health literacy continues to evolve and grow. It seems like almost every day there are new policies, guidelines, research, resources, tools, and technologies. This book, of course, cannot stay up to date with them all. Here are some resources to help you keep learning about health literacy:

- Go to my Health Literacy Consulting Web site at www.healthliteracy .com. There you can sign up for the monthly e-newsletter "What's New in Health Literacy Consulting."
- Listen to my *Health Literacy Out Loud* podcasts at www.healthliteracyoutloud.com. You can subscribe for free to hear them all.
- Visit the Jones & Bartlett Learning Web page at http://go.jblearning.com/HealthLiteracy. There you can learn more and order additional copies of this book.

Thank you for joining me on this journey called health literacy.

Acknowledgments

Health literacy is bigger than any one person, profession, program, or point of view. Whatever our job or setting, we share an awareness about problems associated with miscommunication and misunderstanding. We also share a sense of advocacy and responsibility to communicate in ways that others can understand.

The *Second Edition* of *Health Literacy from A to Z* is only possible thanks to the many people who so graciously shared stories, provided resources, reviewed drafts, offered suggestions, or otherwise helped me all along the way. From A to Z, my most sincere gratitude and appreciation goes to:

Lee Aase, Mary Ann Abrams, Andrea Apter, Elyse Barbell, Karen Baker, Jeff Belkora, Michele Berman, Lisa Bernstein, Kevin Brooks, Jack Bruggeman, Linda Burhansstipanov, Karyn Lynn Buxman, David D. Cella, Carolyn Clancy, John Comings, James (Jim) Conway, Sean Coombs, Sandra Cornett, Ken Crannell, Arthur Culbert, Terry Davis, Cecelia (Ceci) and Leonard (Len) Doak, Bill Dupes, Matthew Ferraguto, Catherine Finn, Valerie Fletcher, Kathleen Friedman, Maro Gartside, Izzy Gesell, Mary Alice Gillispie, Steven Grossman, Andrea Gwosdow, Jane Hammond, Healthwise, Jessica Hennessey, Mark Hochhauser, Charity Hope, George Isham, Lisa M. Jones, Randi Kant, Naomi Karten, Joseph Kimble, Perri Klass, Jennifer Knopf Munafo, Harold Law, Winston Lawrence, Joanne Locke, Winona Love, Michael Mackert, Jeanne McGee, Joan Guthrie Medlen, Phyllis Moir, Jo-Elle Mogerman, Erika Vinograd Osborne, Hilary Osborne, Suzanne O'Connor, Janice (Ginny) Redish, Teresa Reilly, Pamela Katz Ressler, Grace Richards, Audrey Riffenburgh, Stacy Robison, Linda Rohret, Donald Rubin, Rima Rudd, Terry Ruhl, Kathryn A. Sabadosa, Dean Schillinger, Karen Schriver, Domenic Screnci, Mache Seibel, Carolyn I. Speros, Cynthia Stuen, Bita Tabesh, Mark Tatro, Linda Varone, Constanza Villalba, David Walsh, Curt Wands-Bourdoiseau, Adam Weiss, Joe Weisse, Archie Willard, and Joseph Zoske.

Thank you!

About the Author

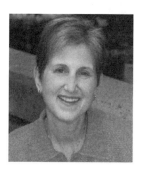

Helen Osborne, MEd, OTR/L
Recognized for her expertise in health literacy, Helen helps health professionals communicate in ways that patients and their families can understand. She does so through a range of consulting, training, and writing services.

Helen is president of Health Literacy Consulting, based in Natick, Massachusetts. She is also the founder of Health Literacy Month, a worldwide campaign to raise awareness about the importance of understandable health information. In addition, Helen produces and hosts the podcast series *Health Literacy Out Loud*.

Helen brings clinical experience, educational training, and patient perspective to all her work. She gives health literacy presentations across the United States and Canada as well as overseas. She also serves as a plain language writer/editor on numerous projects. Several of these have won plain language awards from the National Institutes of Health.

For many years, Helen was a columnist for the Boston Globe Media's *On Call* magazine, writing about patient education and healthcare communication. She is the author of several books, including the award-winning *First Edition* of *Health Literacy from A to Z: Practical Ways to Communicate Your Health Message*—considered by many as the most important health literacy reference today. To learn more about Helen's work, please visit the Health Literacy Consulting Web site at www.healthliteracy.com. You can also listen to her *Health Literacy Out Loud* podcast interviews at www.healthliteracyoutloud.com.

Reviewers

Michael D. Aldridge, MSN, RN, CNS
Assistant Professor of Nursing
Concordia University Texas
Austin, Texas

Su-yan L. Barrow, RDH, MA, MPH
University of Melbourne
Melbourne, Victoria
Australia

Nancy Danou, RN, MSN, CPN
Associate Professor
Viterbo University
La Crosse, Wisconsin

Diane H. Gronefeld, MEd, RT(RM)
Associate Professor, Department of Allied Health
Northern Kentucky University
Highland Heights, Kentucky

Mark Jaffe, DPM, MHSA
Associate Professor
Nova Southeastern University
Fort Lauderdale, Florida

Allison Kabel, PhD
Assistant Professor, Health Sciences Program
School of Health Professions
University of Missouri
Columbia, Missouri

Cindy K. Manjounes, EdD
Department Chair, Healthcare Administration
Lindenwood University
Saint Charles, Missouri

Carol Shenise, MS, RN
Professor
Excelsior College
Albany, New York

Melissa Vosen, PhD
Academic Adviser and Lecturer
College of University Studies and Department of English
North Dakota State University
Fargo, North Dakota

About Health Literacy

Health literacy is about communicating health information clearly and understanding it correctly. Health literacy is relevant at all points along the continuum of care—from wellness and health; to disease prevention and detection; to diagnosis and decision making; to treatment and self-care.

Health information is communicated in many ways. Certainly this includes one-to-one conversations and written materials. Health communication also takes other forms, including Web sites, text messages, podcasts, pictures, phone calls, and classes. Regardless of the form communication takes, the consistent goal is to promote health understanding.

Because health literacy includes the word "literacy," many people assume that it is only a concern for those who cannot read. But this assumption is incorrect. People have difficulty understanding health information for a range of reasons that include literacy, age, disability, language, culture, and emotion. I know. Although I am a well-educated health professional and fluent reader, when a provider tells me upsetting news I tend to "shut down" and, for at least a while, cannot truly understand what the health provider is communicating to me. (Read more about specific populations at "Know Your Audience," starting on page 93.)

WHAT IS THE DEFINITION OF HEALTH LITERACY?

The definition of health literacy is in flux. The most widely used definition in the United States is that health literacy is "the degree to which individuals have the capacity to obtain, process, and understand basic health information and services needed to make appropriate health decisions" (Selden, Zorn, Ratzan, & Parker 2000). While this definition looks at an individual's skills (or perhaps, the lack thereof), others frame health literacy in terms of the literacy demands in the environment of care (Rudd & Anderson 2006). Other definitions focus on populations, not individuals, looking to public health decisions that benefit the community (Freedman et al. 2009). And yet another definition questions whether health literacy is a clinical risk or personal asset (Nutbeam 2008).

My working definition of health literacy is quite general, focusing on outcomes rather than specific places or populations. To me, health literacy is a shared responsibility between patients (or anyone on the receiving end of health communication) and providers (or anyone on the giving end of health communication). Both must communicate in ways the other can understand.

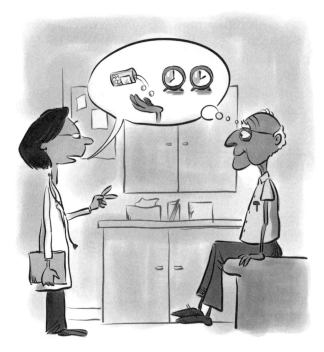

Health Literacy—When Patients and Providers Truly Understand One Another

Source: Illustration by Mark Tatro, Rotate Graphics

WHY, HOW, AND WHEN DID HEALTH LITERACY BEGIN?

Leonard (Len) and Cecelia (Ceci) Doak are widely acknowledged for lead-ing the way when it comes to health literacy. Their award-winning book *Teaching Patients with Low Literacy Skills* was, and still is, an essential how-to guide for communicating clearly with patients.

I asked the Doaks how they got started. They said their interest in health literacy began with their marriage in 1973. At that time, Len was a literacy tutor and Ceci a health educator. As Ceci explains, "When I met Len and he told me he volunteered as a tutor with people who couldn't read and write, I said, 'My heavens! How do people with low literacy skills understand medi-cal advice? What happens when they go to the doctor?' Len replied, 'Often, they don't understand.'"

And so began the Doaks' health literacy journey. Their goal then, as now, is to help health professionals "work around" literacy issues so that patients leave appointments knowing what to do and how to do it (Osborne 2009, March 23).

WHY IS HEALTH LITERACY IMPORTANT NOW?

Health literacy is now at the forefront of many health initiatives. But why? In my opinion, there are several reasons why health literacy matters today:

- *Patients need to understand health information quickly because they have less face-to-face time with their providers.* This includes brief office appoint-ments and short hospitalizations.
- *Patients, along with their family members and other caregivers, are expected to correctly accomplish a wide array of health-related tasks.* These tasks may be complex and unfamiliar, such as using new types of technology or taking medication on time-sensitive schedules.
- *Patients must be active learners.* This includes reading information given to them by providers as well as assessing the credibility and relevance of health information from family and friends, popular media, and the Internet.
- *Patients are increasingly seen as active consumers rather than passive recipients of treatment and care.* Patients today are often asked to make key health decisions and expected to advocate on their own behalf.

And somewhat cynically, I believe that one of the few ways left to reduce healthcare costs is by having patients and families take care of themselves. This requires knowing what to do, how to do it, and why it is important. In other words, this high level of self-care takes a heaping dose of health literacy. Below is an everyday example of the need for health literacy.

Stories from Practice: Health Literacy in Everyday Tasks

Rima Rudd, ScD, Senior Lecturer on Society, Human Development, and Health at the Harvard School of Public Health, has looked at the big picture of health literacy policy as well as assessed everyday tasks that patients must accomplish. In a *Health Literacy Out Loud* podcast, she spoke about the many tasks that compose a "health activity," such as taking medicine.

"When you begin to list out the component tasks of what we sometimes think of as a single activity, you begin to appreciate the sophisticated literacy skills involved. Taking medicine involves multiple tasks. You have to get a prescription filled, bring the medicine home, and be able to read the label. If, as is true for many people, you happen to be taking other medicines, you have to differentiate Medicine A from Medicine B. You really have to read the label with a great deal of care and be able to at least recognize, if not pronounce, the name of the medicine.

"You have to be able to read and comprehend the directions. The directions are often poorly written. Let's say you're told that you need to take this medicine on an empty stomach. That is a jargon term. You have to be able to be familiar with the words of the trade. An empty stomach means not just that you haven't eaten for the past two hours when you take the medicine but that you're not going to eat for another two to three hours. That's not clearly directed.

"Other activities have to do with timing and using a clock. Consider subtracting two hours from 1:30 when you only have a digital clock. You need to use a calendar to note frequency and duration of the prescription. For example, you might take some arthritis medicine only once a week. You will also need to track the time so that you do not run out of medicine. This means that you need to know when you have to get a refill so that you're not skipping a couple of days. As you can see, taking medicine really covers a wide variety of tasks."

Source: Osborne (2009, May 4).

ADVOCATING FOR HEALTH LITERACY

There is a growing movement toward health literacy solutions. In 2010, the United States launched the initiative, *National Action Plan to Improve Health Literacy*. It includes seven goals and numerous suggested strategies that organizations and professions can use to improve health literacy. Goals are to:

1. "Develop and disseminate health and safety information that is accurate, accessible, and actionable.
2. Promote changes in the healthcare system that improve health information, communication, informed decision making, and access to health services.
3. Incorporate accurate, standards-based, and developmentally appropriate health and science information and curricula in child care and education through the university level.
4. Support and expand local efforts to provide adult education, English language instruction, and culturally and linguistically appropriate health information services in the community.
5. Build partnerships, develop guidance, and change policies.
6. Increase basic research and the development, implementation, and evaluation of practices and interventions to improve health literacy.
7. Increase the dissemination and use of evidence-based health literacy practices and interventions" (U.S. Department of Health and Human Services 2010).

As stated in the summary of the *National Action Plan to Improve Health Literacy*, "By focusing on health literacy issues and working together, we can improve the accessibility, quality, and safety of health care; reduce costs; and improve the health and quality of life of millions of people in the United States" (U.S. Department of Health and Human Services, 2010).

Health literacy matters now more than ever. It is up to each of us— whether as patients, providers, or policy makers—to create effective strategies, build sustainable coalitions, and advocate for long-term solutions. I strongly believe that by working together, we indeed can make a long-lasting health literacy difference.

 Health literacy is a shared responsibility between patients (or anyone on the receiving end of health communication) and providers (or anyone on the giving end of health communication). Both must communicate in ways the other can understand.

—Helen Osborne's functional definition of health literacy.

CITATIONS

Doak CC, Doak LG, Root JH. 1996. *Teaching Patients with Low Literacy Skills*. 2nd ed. Philadelphia: J. B. Lippincott. Available at http://www.hsph.harvard.edu/ healthliteracy/resources/doak-book/index.html. Accessed December 30, 2010.

Freedman DA, Bess KD, Tucker HA, Boyd DL, Tuchman AM, Wallston KA. 2009. Public Health Literacy Defined. *American Journal of Preventive Medicine.* 36(5):446–451.

Nutbeam D. 2008. The Evolving Concept of Health Literacy. *Social Science and Medicine.* 67(12):2072–2078.

Osborne H (host). 2009, March 23. Len and Ceci Doak Discuss Health Literacy's Past, Present, and Future [audio podcast]. *Health Literacy Out Loud,* no. 13. Available at http://healthliteracy.com/hlol-doaks. Accessed December 30, 2010.

Osborne H (host). 2009, May 4. Dr. Rima Rudd Talks About the Health Literacy Burden in Healthcare [audio podcast]. *Health Literacy Out Loud,* no. 15. Available at http://www.hlol-rima rudd. Accessed December 30, 2010.

Rudd RE, Anderson JE. 2006. *The Health Literacy Environment of Hospitals and Health Centers: Partners for Action: Making Your Healthcare Facility Literacy-Friendly.* Cambridge, MA: National Center for the Study of Adult Learning and Literacy & Health and Adult Literacy and Learning Initiative, Harvard School of Public Health. Available at http://www.hsph.harvard.edu/healthliteracy/files/healthliteracyenvironment .pdf. Accessed December 29, 2010.

Selden CR, Zorn M, Ratzan S, Parker RM. 2000. *Health Literacy: January 1990 through 1999.* NLM Publication # CBM2000-1. Bethesda, MD: National Library of Medicine. Available at http://www.nlm.nih.gov/archive/20061214/pubs/cbm/ hliteracy.pdf. Accessed June 13, 2011.

U.S. Department of Health and Human Services. 2010. *National Action Plan to Improve Health Literacy.* Available at http://www.health.gov/communication/ HLActionPlan. Accessed December 30, 2010.

Sources to Learn More

American Academy of Health Behavior. 2007. Health Literacy Supplement. *American Journal of Health Behavior.* 31(Suppl. 1). Available at http://www.ajhb.org/ issues/2007/31-s1.htm. Accessed June 13, 2011.

American Medical Association. 2007. *Health Literacy and Patient Safety: Help Patients Understand* [video]. Available at http://www.ama-assn.org/ama/pub/about-ama/ama-foundation/our-programs/public-health/health-literacy-program/ health-literacy-video.page. Accessed April 18, 2011.

CDC (Centers for Disease Control and Prevention). n.d. *Health Literacy for Public Health Professionals* [Web-based training program]. Course number WB1285. Available at http://www2a.cdc.gov/TCEOnline/registration/detailpage .asp?res_id=2074. Accessed June 12, 2010.

CDC (Centers for Disease Control and Prevention). 2011. *Health Literacy: Accurate, Accessible and Actionable Health Information.* Available at http://cdc.gov/ healthliteracy/. Accessed April 20, 2011.

DeWalt DA, Callahan LF, Hawk VH, Broucksou KA, Hink A, Rudd R, Brach C. 2010. *Health Literacy Universal Precautions Toolkit.* Prepared by North Carolina Network Consortium, The Cecil G. Sheps Center for Health Services Research,

The University of North Carolina at Chapel Hill, under Contract No. HHSA290200710014. AHRQ Publication No. 10-0046-EF. Rockville, MD: Agency for Healthcare Research and Quality.

Eichler K, Wieser S, Brügger U. 2009. The Costs of Limited Health Literacy: A Systematic Review. *International Journal of Public Health.* 54(5):313–324.

Harvard School of Public Health. n.d. *Health Literacy Studies.* http://www.hsph .harvard.edu/healthliteracy/. Accessed December 30, 2010.

Health Literacy Consulting, www.healthliteracy.com. Includes Helen Osborne's articles, tips, and a free "What's New" e-newsletter.

Health Literacy Month, www.healthliteracymonth.org. Worldwide campaign to raise awareness about the importance of understandable health information.

Kripalani S, Paasche-Orlow MK, Parker RM, Saha S (eds.). 2006. Health Literacy [Special Issue]. *Journal of General Internal Medicine.* 21(8).

LINCS (Literacy Information and Communication System), Health literacy discussion list. Archives available at http://lincs.ed.gov/pipermail/healthliteracy/2011/ date.html. Accessed January 25, 2011.

Maastricht University, Department of International Health. n.d. *The European Health Literacy Survey.* Available at http://www.health-literacy.eu. Accessed December 30, 2010.

Mayer GG, Villaire M. 2007. *Health Literacy in Primary Care: A Clinician's Guide.* New York: Springer.

National Center for Education Statistics. 2003. *National Assessment of Adult Literacy (NAAL).* Available at http://nces.ed.gov/naal. Accessed December 30, 2010.

Nielsen-Bohlman L, Panzer AM, Kindig DA (eds.). 2004. *Health Literacy: A Prescription to End Confusion.* Washington, DC: National Academies Press.

Olson DP, Windish DM. 2010. Communication Discrepancies Between Physicians and Hospitalized Patients. *Archives of Internal Medicine.* 170(15):1302–1307.

Osborne H (host). 2010, June 8. National Action Plan to Improve Health Literacy [audio podcast]. *Health Literacy Out Loud,* no. 39. Available at http://www .healthliteracy.com/hlol-national-health-literacy-action-plan. Accessed August 25, 2010.

Osborne H (host). 2011, March 22. Health Literacy Milestones and Opportunities [audio podcast]. *Health Literacy Out Loud,* no. 55. Available at http:// healthliteracy.com/hlol-milestones-opportunities. Accessed April 20, 2011.

Parker R, Ratzan SC. 2010. Health Literacy: A Second Decade of Distinction for Americans. *Journal of Health Communication: International Perspectives.* 15(S2):20–33.

Rudd R, Kirsch I, Yamamoto K, 2004. *Literacy and Health in America.* Princeton, NJ: Center for Global Assessment, Policy Information Center, Research and Development, Educational Testing Services.

Rudd RE. 2010. Improving Americans' Health Literacy. *New England Journal of Medicine.* 363(24):2283–2285.

Rudd RE, Zobel EK, Fanta CH, Surkan P, Rodriguez-Louis J, Valderrama Y, Daltroy LH. 2004. Asthma in Plain Language. *Health Promotion Practice.* 5(3):334–340.

Schwartzberg JG, VanGeest JB, Wang CC (eds.). 2005. *Understanding Health Literacy: Implications for Medicine and Public Health.* Chicago: American Medical Association Press.

The Joint Commission. 2010. *Advancing Effective Communication, Cultural Competence, and Patient- and Family-Centered Care: A Roadmap for Hospitals.* Oakbrook Terrace, IL: The Joint Commission. Available at http://www .jointcommission.org/assets/1/6/ARoadmapforHospitalsfinalversion727 .pdf. Accessed May 19, 2011.

U.S. Department of Health and Human Services, Health Resources and Services Administration (HRSA). n.d. *Unified Health Communication (UHC): Addressing Health Literacy, Cultural Competency, and Limited English Proficiency* [online training program]. Available at http://www.hrsa.gov/publichealth/healthliteracy/ Accessed June 12, 2010.

Zarcadoolas C, Pleasant AF, Greer DS. 2006. *Advancing Health Literacy: A Framework for Understanding and Action.* San Francisco: Jossey-Bass.

Assessing Health Literacy

Is it important to assess how well your patients can read, understand, and act on health information? If so, what assessment tool would you use to measure these skills? Would you use this tool to assess individuals or the overall level of your patient population? And if it is important to make these assessments, and you had the correct tool and knew which patients to test, how would doing so make a difference in your practice?

Clinicians, health educators, and others responsible for day-to-pay patient communication are grappling with questions like these. But there does not yet seem to be consensus on best practices when it comes to assessing health literacy. Here is a brief look at reasons to, and not to, routinely assess health literacy skills in clinical practice.

Reasons to routinely assess health literacy skills. Some professionals assert that knowing the level of each patient's health literacy skills will guide the choice of teaching methods and materials. Here is an example:

> Jane reads at a fourth-grade level. She is asked to fill out a health history form before seeing her new primary care provider. Jane has learned from experience that it is easiest to simply check "no" for all questions on the form about illnesses and allergies. This way, there are fewer follow-up questions. But it turns out that Jane's strategy has costly consequences, as her provider unknowingly prescribes a medication to which she is allergic.

Those who advocate for routinely assessing health literacy might argue that if Jane's provider knew that she could barely read, then he or she could offer alternatives, such as a simply written health history that includes graphics, or someone to assist Jane in completing the form.

Reasons not to routinely assess health literacy skills. Other professionals dispute the value of routine health literacy screening, arguing that formal assessments can do more harm than good. They feel that patients may perceive formal assessments as literacy tests, which, in turn, can promote feelings of anxiety and shame.

Rather than assessing individual patients, many providers advocate for universal precautions when it comes to health communication. This includes routinely watching for "red flags" of communication problems (see "Informal Ways to Assess Health Literacy" on page 12), asking patients how they like to learn, offering a range of print and non-print educational tools, and consistently using the teach-back method to confirm understanding. (Read more in "Universal Design in Communication" starting on page 209 and "Confirming Understanding" starting on page 35.)

Stories from Practice: A New Reader's View of Health Literacy Assessments

Archie Willard refers to himself as a "new reader," someone who learned to read as an adult. Willard is an ardent, articulate health literacy advocate and has chaired several health literacy conferences for fellow new readers. Here is his opinion about literacy testing in healthcare settings:

"There are those in the medical field who feel literacy testing should be done to receive medical attention. From your viewpoint it looks like a good idea, but you need to look through the eyes of the person who has literacy problems. As a dyslexic and an adult learner with reading problems, I speak for many other adult learners.

"We hate having to take another written literacy test. People with other kinds of handicaps are not continually asked to expose their weaknesses to whatever degree they are handicapped. There is no physical pain in taking a written test, but when we have to there is a lot of frustration inside each of us. We grew up feeling humiliated because we had poor literacy skills and now we are adults. More written tests are seen as another step backward for us and it turns us away."

Source: Literacy Information and Communication System (2004).

STRATEGIES, IDEAS, AND SUGGESTIONS

Here are some ideas to consider:

Use formal health literacy assessment tools. There is a growing array of tools to assess health literacy. Some focus primarily on reading or word recognition skills, while others include common healthcare tasks, such as numeracy. Some tools need to be administered by professionals, and others by trained staff. And there is even an assessment tool that patients can complete on their own. Tools are also being developed for specific populations, diagnoses, and languages. Here are some health literacy assessment tools:

- **BEHKA—HIV Version (Brief Estimate of Health Knowledge and Action).** This tool is a brief, eight-item assessment of HIV treatment knowledge and action. Researchers report, "This set of knowledge and action capacity may better represent health literacy for HIV patients than more general measures of reading ability or health vocabulary" (Osborn, Davis, Bailey, & Wolf 2010).
- **METER (Medical Term Recognition Test).** This is a short, self-administered measure of health literacy. Patients are given a list of items and asked to check those they recognize as actual words. Researchers report that the "METER is administered as quickly as the REALM [described below], with minimal instructions and involvement of practitioners and it correlates highly with the REALM" (Rawson et al. 2010).
- **NVS (Newest Vital Sign).** Patients answer six standardized questions about a sample ice cream label. For example, "If you eat the entire container, how many calories will you eat?" The NVS takes about three minutes to administer and is available in English or Spanish. Researchers report that the NVS is "a reliable and accurate measure of literacy with high sensitivity for detecting persons with limited literacy" (Weiss et al. 2005).
- **REALM (Rapid Estimate of Adult Literacy in Medicine).** This well-regarded and often-used tool looks at recognition of written health words. The REALM asks patients to pronounce 66 words ranging in difficulty from "fat" to "impetigo." It is easy to administer and provides grade-level scores for people who read below a ninth-grade level (Davis et al. 1993).
- **SAHL–S&E (Short Assessment of Health Literacy–Spanish and English).** This tool combines a word recognition test (adapted from the REALM) along with a comprehension test using multi-choice questions. It can be given in Spanish or English. Researchers report it "could be used to screen for low health literacy among Spanish and English speakers" (Lee et al. 2010).

- **SOS.** This mnemonic device includes three components: (1) educational attainment ("the person's schooling is . . . "), (2) self-rated reading ability ("the person's opinion of his or her reading ability is . . . "), and (3) help needed when reading ("when the person reads health-related materials, support is . . . "). Researchers propose using the SOS "to help clinicians wishing to individualize patient education" (Jeppesen, Coyle, & Miser 2009).
- **Single-question screening tool.** Researchers looked at questions designed to help identify patients with limited or marginal health literacy skills. They report that the question with most utility was, "How confident are you filling out medical forms by yourself?" The authors of this study write that "the use of a single question to screen for limited literacy could obviate the need for more formal health literacy assessments in clinical settings" (Wallace, Rogers, Roskos, Holiday, & Weiss 2006).
- **TOFHLA (Test of Functional Health Literacy in Adults)** and **S-TOFHLA** (shortened version). Each of these assessment tools includes a series of health-related reading tasks that measure numeracy and reading comprehension. These well-regarded assessment tools have been used in research studies for many years (Parker, Baker, Williams, & Nurss 1995).
- **TOFHLA-SPR.** This Spanish-language version of the TOFHLA was adapted for use in Puerto Rico. In a research article, the authors conclude, "Findings support the need to tailor instruments within a language and to different contexts which would make the instrument unique because it would take into account the cultural nuances of that language" (Rivero-Méndez et al. 2010).

Use informal ways to assess health literacy. Many practitioners and adult learners recommend that, in lieu of formal assessments, clinicians learn to recognize "red flags" of health literacy problems. Such red flags include when patients:

- Consistently have "headaches" or chronically "forget" their eyeglasses when asked to perform reading tasks.
- Often say their hands hurt and will fill out paperwork at home.
- Regularly ask family members, friends, or others to read written materials aloud.
- Identify medications by looking at the pills themselves, rather than reading prescription labels.
- Ask a lot of questions about topics already covered in handouts and brochures.

Just because someone has a headache, an achy hand, or asks a lot of questions does not necessarily mean that he or she has limited health literacy. But in my opinion, noticing these red flags is a good place to start your assessment.

 Is it important to assess how well your patients can read, understand, and act on health information? If so, what assessment tool would you use to measure these skills? How would doing so make a difference in your practice?

CITATIONS

Davis TC, Long SW, Jackson RH, Mayeaux EJ, George RB, Murphy PW, Crouch MA. 1993. Rapid Estimate of Adult Literacy in Medicine: A Shortened Screening Instrument. *Family Medicine.* 25(6):391–395.

Jeppesen KM, Coyle JD, Miser WF. 2009. Screening Questions to Predict Limited Health Literacy: A Cross-Sectional Study of Patients with Diabetes Mellitus. *Annals of Family Medicine.* 7(1):24–31.

Lee SD, Stucky BD, Lee JY, Rozier RG, Bender DE. 2010. Short Assessment of Health Literacy—Spanish and English: A Comparable Test of Health Literacy for Spanish and English Speakers. *Health Services Research.* 45(4): 1105–1120.

LINCS (Literacy Information and Communication System). 2004. Health Literacy discussion list. Available at http://lincs.ed.gov/mailman/listinfo/Healthliteracy/. Accessed April 20, 2011.

Osborn CY, Davis TC, Bailey SC, Wolf MS. 2010. Health Literacy in the Context of HIV Treatment: Introducing the Brief Estimate of Health Knowledge and Action (BEHKA)—HIV Version. *AIDS and Behavior.* 14(1):181–188.

Parker RM, Baker DW, Williams MV, Nurss JR. 1995. The Test of Functional Health Literacy in Adults: A New Instrument for Measuring Patients' Literacy Skills. *Journal of General Internal Medicine.* 10(10):537–541.

Rawson KA, Gunstad J, Hughes J, Spitznagel MB, Potter V, Waechter D, Rosneck J. 2010. The METER: A Brief, Self-Administered Measure of Health Literacy. *Journal of General Internal Medicine.* 25(1):67–71.

Rivero-Méndez M, Suárez E, Solís-Báez SS, Hernández G, Cordero W, Vázquez I, et al. 2010. Internal Consistency of the Spanish Health Literacy Test (TOFHLA-SPR) for Puerto Rico. *Puerto Rico Health Sciences Journal.* 29(1):49–53.

Wallace LS, Rogers ES, Roskos SE, Holiday DB, Weiss BD. 2006. Brief Report: Screening Items to Identify Patients with Limited Health Literacy Skills. *Journal of General Internal Medicine.* 21(8):874–877.

Weiss BD, Mays MZ, Martz W, Castro KM, DeWalt DA, Pignone MP, et al. 2005. Quick Assessment of Literacy in Primary Care: The Newest Vital Sign. *Annals of Family Medicine.* 3(6):514–522.

Sources to Learn More

Dowse R, Lecoko L, Ehlers M. 2010. Applicability of the REALM Health Literacy Test to an English Second-Language South African Population. *Pharmacy World and Science.* 32(4):464–471.

Elliott VS. 2008, June 2. *Experts Debate Value of Assessing Health Literacy.* Amednews .com. Available at http://www.ama-assn.org/amednews/2008/06/02/hlsd0602 .htm. Accessed April 16, 2011.

Johnson K, Weiss BD. 2008. How Long Does It Take to Assess Literacy Skills in Clinical Practice? *Journal of the American Board of Family Medicine.* 21(3):211–214.

Osborne H. 2007. In Other Words . . . Screening for Health Literacy Using the Newest Vital Sign. *On Call.* Available at http://www.healthliteracy.com/newest-vital-sign Accessed September 9, 2010.

Osborne H (host). 2008, October 20. Archie Willard Talks About Struggling to Read [audio podcast]. *Health Literacy Out Loud,* no. 3. Available at http:// healthliteracy.com/hlol-archie-willard. Accessed July 22, 2010.

Ryan JG, Leguen F, Weiss BD, Albury S, Jennings T, Velez F, Salibi N. 2007. Will Patients Agree to Have Their Literacy Skills Assessed in Clinical Practice? *Health Education Research.* 23(4):603–611.

Shah LC, West P, Bremmeyr K, Savoy-Moore RT. 2010. Health Literacy Instrument in Family Medicine: The "Newest Vital Sign" Ease of Use and Correlates. *Journal of the American Board of Family Medicine.* 23(2):195–203.

Assessing Readability with Grade Level Formulas

STARTING POINTS

Many health writers say their materials are easy to read and suitable for readers of average skills, or below. When I ask how they determine this, writers often talk about measuring readability with grade-level formulas (also called "readability assessment tools" or "readability formulas").

I cringe if this is the only way they assess readability, especially when writers rely solely on formulas within word-processing programs. Although arguably better than nothing, to me (and many others) such formulas are an imperfect and incomplete way to assess readability. Here are some reasons why:

- Some of the most commonly used reading grade–level formulas (including the Fry and the SMOG, discussed later in this chapter) were designed many years ago to help teachers select textbooks for students. These formulas were never intended to measure the readability of health materials written for adults.
- More than 100 factors impact how readable any given document is, including its sentence length, word choice, organization, tone, layout, use of illustrations, and relevance to readers. But most reading grade–level formulas measure just a few of these factors. Commonly, they calculate readability based on the average number of words in sentences and the average number of syllables in words. Nonetheless, research shows that the length of sentences and length of words do

impact reading difficulty the most, says Audrey Riffenbugh, MA, a specialist in plain language and readability and president of Plain Language Works, LLC.

- Studies have shown that among the general public, adults read, "on the average, about five grade levels lower than the last year of school completed" (Doak, Doak, & Root 1996, p. 28). This means that someone with a high school education would likely have difficulty reading materials written above a seventh-grade level.

- Readability formulas are just that—formulas. By looking at punctuation (such as periods), a formula might determine that this statement is three sentences, not one: "Dr. Smith said I should call if my child has a temperature of 100.2." And formulas do not take word order into account. In fact, these are assessed at the same reading level: "The order of words doesn't matter at all" and "All at matter doesn't words of order the."

Despite these drawbacks, reading grade–level formulas are beneficial in that they are objective, easy to use, and the scores almost always get people's attention. I often use such formulas at the beginning and end of plain-language projects to confirm that I made significant improvements. You can assess readability by hand or by computer.

STRATEGIES, IDEAS, AND SUGGESTIONS

Some helpful strategies are listed here:

Assess readability "by hand" (with pencil and paper). The SMOG (Simplified Measurement of Gobbledygook) and the Fry readability formula are two well-regarded reading grade–level tools that can be done by hand. While both give grade-level scores, they calculate them in different ways. The SMOG counts all words with three or more syllables in three 10-sentence passages. The Fry formula looks at the number of syllables and sentences in three 100-word passages. You can find detailed instructions for these and other readability tools on numerous Internet Web sites and writing guides.

Honestly, I like assessing readability by hand. I find the SMOG and Fry easy and quick to use; I can use these formulas with paper documents as well as computer files. I can also decide for myself whether a group of words is a complete sentence, a sentence fragment, or simply a title. And I especially like seeing problem areas. For instance, with the SMOG you circle all multisyllabic words (words with three or more syllables) and so can quickly see which words to change.

Example of Counting Multisyllabic Words by Using the SMOG

Directions for using the SMOG say to count all multisyllabic words (with three or more syllables, including those that are hyphenated) in a 10-sentence passage. Do this for three passages, and then total the number to find the reading grade level on a SMOG chart. Here is one of many places online to find a SMOG chart: http://www.sph .emory.edu/WELLNESS/reading.html.

I used the 10 sentences above, starting with "The SMOG . . ." and ending with ". . . to change." Here are the 30 multisyllabic words that I found:

> Simplified, measurement, gobbledygook, readability, formula, well-regarded, grade-level, grade-level, calculate, different, syllables, 10-sentence, passages, formula, syllables, sentences, 100-word, passages, instructions, readability, numerous, Internet, assessing, readability, formulas, documents, computer, especially, multisyllabic, syllables.

Example of Counting Syllables for the Fry

The directions are to count all syllables in three 100-word passages. You also need to count the number of sentences in those 100 words, to the nearest tenth of a sentence. Do this three times, and then average the syllable scores as well as the sentence scores. You can then use these numbers to find the reading grade level on a Fry graph. Here is one of many online sources for the Fry graph: http://www .idph.state.ia.us/health_literacy/common/pdf/tools/fry.pdf.

Based on some sentences above, here is what syllable count starts to look like:

> Hon-est-ly, I like ass-ess-ing read-a-bil-it-y by hand. I find the Fry and SMOG eas-y and quick to use. I can use these form-u-las with pa-per doc-u-ments as well as com-put-er fil-es. I can al-so de-cide for my-self wheth-er a group of words is a com-plete sen-tence, a sen-tence frag-ment, or simp-ly a ti-tle. And I es-pec-ial-ly like see-ing pro-blem a-re-as. For in-stance, with the SMOG you cir-cle . . .

Stories from Practice: Prepare Text to Get Meaningful Results

I interviewed Audrey Riffenburgh of Plain Language Works, for an article about assessing readability. To get meaningful results with formulas, she reminds writers of guidelines given by the SMOG and Fry about how to prepare the text:

- When possible, choose passages of text that are sufficiently long, ideally with at least 30 sentences or 300 words. If the document you are evaluating is quite long, then assess at least three passages that represent the entire document—one each from the beginning, middle, and end.
- No matter the length of your document, avoid using the first and last sentences, as these are often quite different from the reading level of the rest of the text.

Riffenburgh advocates also preparing text in these ways:

- Remove headings, titles, subtitles, and bullet points. This way, the computer does not give artificially low scores by counting headings and word fragments as complete sentences.
- Take out mid-sentence periods that might be part of an abbreviation or number, such as "Dr." or "100.2." You need to do this because most computer-based assessments are programmed to recognize sentences as groups of words ending with a period, question mark, or exclamation.
- Be cautious not to overinterpret the results. Reading grade-level scores are accurate only by plus or minus one and a half grade levels. This means that when a score drops from 7.3 to 6.8, the document is not necessarily easier to read. Results may vary depending on which formula you use. For example, the Fry formula often scores materials one to two grade levels lower than the SMOG.

Sources: Osborne (2000); Riffenburgh (2011).

Assess readability by computer. Many word processing programs include readability formulas within spelling/grammar check tools. Admittedly, these are fast and easy to use. But there are several limitations, including how these formulas count words and sentences. For instance, formulas may be programmed to count all dots as periods that end sentences (which is not always the case). Or have strict rules about syllables, such as determining incorrectly that the word "people" has three syllables because of the two vowels next to each other.

Assess readability with specially designed software and online tools. My preference when assessing readability by computer is to use software designed for this purpose. In a recent search, I found a dazzling array of readability software and online assessment tools, tests, and calculators. Two readability programs that I like to use are:

- Readability Calculations or Readability Plus, from Micro Power & Light Co. (for PC or Macintosh), http://www.micropowerandlight .com/rd.html.
- Readability Studio (for PC), from OleanderSoftware, http://www .oleandersolutions.com/readabilitystudio.html.

Follow, Do Not Fiddle with, Readability Rules

An area of dispute about readability formulas is whether it is okay to amend the rules and count repetitive, yet necessary, multisyllabic words (like "diabetes") only once instead of each time they appear in the text. While I appreciate that fiddling with these formulas may lower the reading grade level, in my opinion this method can cause as many problems as it solves. For example, once you change this rule, you must create a new one about which multisyllabic words to count. Instead, my method is to follow all the formula's rules but mention in a summary report why the grade-level score is as high as it is.

Explore other ways to assess readability. In addition to using reading grade-level formulas, I advocate using checklists and getting feedback from readers.

- **Checklists.** Checklists can be used throughout the writing process to objectively and subjectively assess a document's strengths, weaknesses, and areas to revise. You can rate content, design, organization, language, tone, appearance, graphics, cultural appropriateness, and other criteria using simple scales (such as "yes/no" or a rating from 1 to 3). One well-regarded checklist is the SAM (Suitability of Assessment of Materials) (Doak, Doak, and Root 1996).

- **Testing materials with readers.** Most health literacy experts agree that the best way to know whether documents are truly easy to read is by asking for feedback from readers representing the intended audience. For example, if you are writing about issues affecting older adults, then you might ask for feedback from members of a local senior center. From your first idea to final draft, those representing your audience are the true experts about a document's relevance, appeal, and readability. In my opinion, that's the best assessment of all. (Read more in "Confirming Understanding: Feedback," starting on page 35.)

 Although arguably better than nothing, to me (and many others) reading grade-level formulas are an imperfect and incomplete way to assess readability.

CITATIONS

Doak C, Doak L, & Root J. 1996. *Teaching Patients with Low Literacy Skills.* Philadelphia: J. B. Lippincott. Available at http://www.hsph.harvard.edu/healthliteracy/resources/doak-book/. Accessed April 13, 2011.

Osborne H. 2000. In Other Words . . . Assessing Readability . . . Rules for Playing the Numbers Game. *On Call.* 3(12):38–39. Available at http://www.healthliteracy.com/assessing-readability. Accessed August 5, 2010.

Riffenburgh A. 2011. Personal communication.

SOURCES TO LEARN MORE

Armbruster BB, Osborn JH, Davison AI. 1985. Readability Formulas May Be Dangerous to Your Textbooks. *Educational Leadership.* 18–20.

Chall JS. 1995. *Readability Revisited: The New Dale-Chall Readability Formula.* Cambridge, MA: Brookline Books/Lumen Editions.

European Commission. 2009, January 12. *Guideline on the Readability of the Labelling and Package Leaflet of Medicinal Products for Human Use.* European Medicines Agency, Revision 1. Available at http://ec.europa.eu/health/files/eudralex/vol-2/c/2009_01_12_readability_guideline_final_en.pdf. Accessed April 13, 2011.

Gibson M, Hochhauser M. 2010. Readability Testing: European Performance vs. USA Formulas. *SoCRA Source: A Publication of the Society of Clinical Research Associates.* 64:69–71.

Gilliam B, Pena SC, Mountain L. 1980. The Fry Graph Applied to Spanish Readability. *Reading Teacher.* 33(4):426–431.

Hochhauser M. 2008, February. Consent Form Readability and Grade Level Are Not the Same. *SoCRA Source: A Publication of the Society of Clinical Research Associates.* 55:35–36.

McLaughlin GH. 1974. Temptations of the Flesch. *Instructional Science.* 2(4):367–384.

MedlinePlus. 2011. *How to Write Easy-to-Read Health Materials.* Available at http://www.nlm.nih.gov/medlineplus/etr.html. Accessed August 5, 2010. Includes links to readability assessment tools as well as readability software programs.

Osborne H (host). 2010, June 29. Assessing Readability in the European Union (EU) [audio podcast]. *Health Literacy Out Loud,* no. 40. Available at http://www.healthliteracy.com/hlol-assessing-readability-in-eu. Accessed August 5, 2010.

Rugimbana R, Patel C. 1996. The Application of the Marketing Concept in Textbook Selection: Using the Cloze Procedure. *Journal of Marketing Education.* 18(1):14–20.

Stevens KC. 1980. Readability Formulae and McCall-Crabbs Standard Test Lessons in Reading. *Reading Teacher.* 33(4):413–415.

U.S. Department of Health & Human Services, Centers for Medicare & Medicaid Services, by Jeanne McGee of McGee & Evers Consulting. 2010. Toolkit Part 7: Using Readability Formulas: A Cautionary Note. *Toolkit for Making Written Material Clear and Effective.* Available at http://www.cms.gov/WrittenMaterialsToolkit/09_ToolkitPart07.asp#TopOfPage. Accessed January 3, 2011.

Business Side of Health Literacy

Those of us on the front lines of health communication need little convincing that health literacy matters. Almost every day we learn of medical errors, hospital readmissions, compromised health status, or other costly outcomes caused, at least in part, by miscommunication and misunderstanding.

Several studies show the high costs of such misunderstandings. An international study found that "on the health system level, the additional costs of limited HL [health literacy] range from 3 to 5% of the total healthcare cost per year. On the patient level, the additional expenditures per year per person with limited HL compared to persons with adequate HL range from US $143 to $7,798" (Eichler, Wieser, & Brügger 2009).

But few studies look at the economic benefits of health literacy. In my opinion we need more research on this topic so as to make a compelling and convincing business case about why health literacy matters. With cost and benefit data, health literacy advocates could frame health literacy issues in ways that resonate with administrators, funders, policy makers, government officials, and others authorized to allocate resources.

Beyond making the case for health literacy, programs also need to aim for sustainability. From a business standpoint, this means that organizations have the resources to continue in the long term and pay for needed staff, marketing, and programs or services. As a consultant to Health Literacy Missouri, David Walsh knows a lot about doing just that. He helped Health

Literacy Missouri develop its long-term vision and sustainable business plan. Below are some of his strategies and suggestions.

STRATEGIES, IDEAS, AND SUGGESTIONS

Here are some strategies you might find useful (Osborne 2010):

Think in terms of business and finances. Health care today is a multi-billion-dollar operation with hospitals, healthcare centers, insurance companies, and doctors thinking about the financial side. Walsh offers health literacy initiatives this advice: "Put yourself in your partner's shoes and think of how they're looking at the operation. A lot of discussions come down to the financial side. It's really the money that allows hospitals and healthcare organizations to provide the highest level of care, to have the funds to do cutting-edge research, and have the resources to be their best."

Use business language. Just as healthcare practitioners expect patients and families to be fluent in medical language, business people want others to understand and use their acronyms, jargon, and industry-specific terms. Here are three very common business terms:

- **Return on investment (ROI).** In terms of health literacy, ROI often has to do with financial benefit (in terms of "net" profit or "bottom line") or mission benefit (meeting goals of an organization's strategic plan).
- **Profit and loss (P&L).** Profit is important to any business or initiative, regardless if it is a for-profit or nonprofit entity. Walsh explains that profit is not a bad thing or a dirty word. "Profit allows organizations to do what they set out to do. In the case of healthcare companies, it is to provide higher levels and better care for their patients," says Walsh.
- **For-profit and not-for-profit.** The distinction between these terms is mostly about tax regulation. In a for-profit business, excess income goes to its shareholders. In a not-for-profit business, profit is invested back into the organization's mission.

Build a team that includes allies and champions. It takes a team to advance most good causes, including health literacy. Recruit "allies" and "champions" to voice support from within, and outside, your organization. Allies and champions often are respected leaders whose support is valued by those at all levels of an organization, association, or community.

Team members may include lawyers who can anticipate roadblocks and help avoid problems, financial advisers to help "crunch" numbers, and a wide range of others, including healthcare administrators, researchers, professors, business executives, community agency directors, government leaders, patients, and the general public.

Stories from Practice: A Visible and Credible Health Literacy Champion

George J. Isham, MD, is Chief Health Officer and Plan Medical Director for HealthPartners Health Plan in Minneapolis, Minnesota. He also chairs the Institute of Medicine's (IOM) Roundtable on Health Literacy. Dr. Isham is a highly visible and credible health literacy champion.

In a *Health Literacy Out Loud* podcast, Dr. Isham spoke of the need to frame health literacy economics in terms of effectiveness and efficiency. He describes "effectiveness" as incorporating health literacy lessons into acute care as well as preventive services. He describes "efficiency" as making all levels of staff aware of health literacy and teaching them easy-to-use communication strategies to help avoid illnesses, lower costs, and reach the goals of quality care and good health outcomes.

As Dr. Isham says in the podcast, "What has surprised me is that there is so much opportunity to improve health care by paying attention to this topic."

Source: Osborne (2009, April 13).

Create a business plan. Regardless of whether you are proposing a health literacy project, building a community coalition, or creating an entirely new business entity, start with a business plan. Here are some key components:

- **Define your purpose and goals.** State clearly the products, services, or programs you plan to deliver. Walsh advises, "Make an effort to focus in on what you really want to do. It's better to provide a couple of programs or services really well rather than trying to offer too much or too many." Look outside your business for key marketplace "drivers." For instance, if you are starting a hospital-based health literacy initiative, then you might want to offer programs aimed at reducing errors or increasing patient satisfaction.

- **Know your primary audience or target market.** Be clear about the people you serve. Then learn as much about them as you can. For example, planning should be quite different if you are building a community coalition to serve adult literacy students, homebound seniors, or teenagers at risk for obesity.
- **Identify needed resources.** What do you need to accomplish your goals? Think about your project's many components, including staff (paid, volunteer, or both), technology, and supplies. I know that as the sole proprietor of a consulting business, I'm amazed at how much "stuff" I always seem to need.
- **Find funding sources.** There are two basic types of funding sources for most health literacy programs. One funding source is "contributed support," referring to private donations, foundations, research grants, and the like. The other source is "fee for service," referring to money that comes in from providing expertise, training, or other services. Many health literacy efforts build on both types of funding.
- **Define measures of success.** All good business plans have milestones and timelines for goals to accomplish. Walsh advises revisiting these goals at least once a year. "Whether or not you feel you're doing great or doing bad, you should always go back and say, 'Okay, here's what we said we're going to do. Now let's see how we did against those goals.'"

 With cost and benefit data, health literacy advocates could frame health literacy issues in ways that resonate with administrators, funders, policy makers, government officials, or others authorized to allocate resources.

CITATIONS

Eichler K, Wieser S, Brügger U. 2009. The Costs of Limited Health Literacy: A Systematic Review. *International Journal of Public Health.* 54(5):313–324.

Osborne H (host). 2009, April 13. Talking About the Economic Side of Health Literacy [audio podcast]. *Health Literacy Out Loud,* no. 14. Available at http://healthliteracy.com/hlol-health-literacy-economics. Accessed April 20, 2011.

Osborne H (host). 2010, January 5. Making a Business Case to Move Health Literacy Forward [audio podcast]. *Health Literacy Out Loud,* no. 30. Available at http://healthliteracy.com/hlol-business-case. Accessed April 20, 2011.

Sources to Learn More

Isham GJ, Halvorson GC. 2003. *Epidemic of Care: A Call for Safer, Better, and More Accountable Health Care.* San Francisco, CA: Jossey-Bass.

National Academy of Sciences, Institute of Medicine. 2011. *Roundtable on Health Literacy.* Available at http://www.iom.edu/Activities/PublicHealth/HealthLiteracy.aspx. Accessed April 16, 2011.

Nielsen-Bohlman L, Panzer AM, Kindig DA (eds.). 2004. *Health Literacy: A Prescription to End Confusion.* Committee on Health Literacy. Board on Neuroscience and Behavioral Health. Institute of Medicine of the National Academies. Washington, DC: National Academies Press.

Osborne H. 2006, September/October. In Other Words . . . Making a Bottom-Line Case for Health Literacy. *On Call.* Available at http://www.healthliteracy.com/bottom-line. Accessed April 20, 2011.

Communicating When Patients Feel Scared, Sick, and Overwhelmed

STARTING POINTS

When patients and providers fail to communicate adequately, both parties potentially suffer. Providers need to present information about new diagnoses, treatment options, and self-care instructions. Patients need to describe their symptoms, ask questions, and express opinions about treatment and care. And both need to listen closely, respond thoughtfully, and remember clearly what each other just said.

This type of back-and-forth communication is hard to do, but it is often more so when patients are feeling sick, scared, and overwhelmed. Here are strategies about how providers can help patients—and how patients can help themselves—when communicating about health.

STRATEGIES, IDEAS, AND SUGGESTIONS

Strategies for Providers

Here are suggestions that providers can put into practice:

Appreciate why communication can be hard for patients. Many patients find it difficult to participate in health conversations. They may fear that providers won't like them if they ask too many questions. They may feel ashamed to admit not understanding certain medical terms or concepts. And, as I and many others know, when faced with health challenges, it's exceedingly difficult to think quickly and communicate clearly when feeling vulnerable and exposed. In other words, it's very hard to communicate when naked.

Honor the patient's experience. Patients are, or after a new diagnosis will soon be, experts on what it's like to live with their disease or condition. Find out how much information patients want to know and how willing they are to be involved in treatment and care. Decide together what to discuss. You most likely can accommodate both their priorities and yours, but perhaps in a different order than you expected. (Read more in "Decision Aids and Shared Decision-Making," starting on page 45.)

Help patients ask questions. Encourage patients to anticipate questions they want to ask. You can help by giving patients tools like notepads to write down their questions about diagnoses, treatment, and medical instructions. Make sure to leave room for patients to also write down your answers. And please provide a pen, pencil, and clipboard or other hard writing surface, as these items are increasingly hard to find in examining rooms today. (Read more in "Question Asking," starting on page 167.)

Acknowledge articles and printouts that patients bring to you. Patients today may come to appointments already somewhat informed; they may have heard or read about their illnesses or medications in the newspaper, on television, on the Internet, or in direct-to-consumer advertising. Let patients know that you value their efforts and are open to their suggestions and questions. But also discuss the fact that sometimes information like this is incorrect, biased, or sensationalized. (Read more in "General Public: Talking with Patients About What They Learn from the Media," starting on page 73.)

Confirm that you and your patients understand each other. Pause periodically after key points and again at the end of appointments or conversations and ask patients to tell you, in their own words, what you just discussed. Assume responsibility by starting with a statement like, "I just want to make sure I explained this clearly. Please tell me how you will . . . " (Read more in "Confirming Understanding: Teach-Back Technique," starting on page 41.)

Help patients learn more. Make it easy for patients to learn as much as they want to know. Prepare lists of credible resources, including books, articles, Web sites, hotlines, and associations. You might also want to let patients know about blogs devoted to helping patients be more activated and engaged patients. (Read more in "Technology: Blogs and Other Social Media," starting on page 193.)

Stories from Practice: Communicating When Naked—My Perspective as a Patient

Talking about health and other medical matters had always been easy for me. As an occupational therapist and health-literacy consultant, I felt confident and in charge of conversations no matter which professional hat I was wearing. But after a routine mammogram turned out not to be so routine, I felt more than hatless. I felt naked. Now I had to communicate not as a provider or consultant, but as a patient.

The diagnosis was DCIS (ductal carcinoma in situ, a very early stage of breast cancer). Ironically, this was a condition I knew a good deal about. The year before, I helped write the National Cancer Institute booklet *Surgery Options for Women with Early Stage Breast Cancer*. But as a patient, I became easily overwhelmed when talking with doctors about my diagnosis and treatment options. Since the conversations concerned me directly, I was often so flooded with emotion that I had trouble thinking and remembering.

Eventually conversations got easier and I learned what I needed to know and do.

But I learned something else, too. The biggest, most profound and important lesson I learned is that health literacy truly matters—to all of us who are, or ever will be, on either side of health conversations.

Source: Osborne (2006).

Strategies for Patients

Here are some ideas that patients might want to try (Osborne 2005, 2006):

Take note of your symptoms. Keep track of when your symptoms started, how often they occur, and how long each episode lasts. Describe your symptoms in ways that help the provider understand. For instance, you could describe the intensity of pain using a combination of numbers and words. Even if your provider doesn't ask, you can rate the pain on a scale of 1 (no pain) to 10 (worst pain ever). And you can supplement this rating with descriptive words about the pain, such as "achy," "burning," "stabbing," "stiff," "tingly," "sore," or "annoying."

Invite family members or friends to act as advocates. It can be extra hard to advocate for yourself when feeling vulnerable, scared, overwhelmed, or ill. If you can anticipate that conversations might be difficult, consider inviting a family member or friend to help by taking notes, voicing concerns, and remembering what was said. If this person cannot be present at important meetings, try to arrange other ways for that person to be involved, such as saying to your provider, "My son wants to talk with you. When is a good time for him to call?" Saying something like this not only creates a follow-up plan but also gives permission for your provider to speak with this person.

Overcome communication barriers. If you use hearing aids or eyeglasses, bring them to your appointments. Tell your provider if he or she is speaking too softly, if the print size in written materials is too small to read, or if there are words, concepts, and numbers you do not fully understand.

Learn only as much as you want to know. What surprised me the most when dealing with a serious diagnosis was that, for at least a while, I did not want a lot of "outside" Web site or book information. I've come to appreciate that there is no right or wrong amount. While I was comforted by limited amounts of outside information, many others find it helpful to research as much as they can. My advice to patients is to learn only as much as you want to know now. Later, you can always find out more.

Create your own medical record. Just as health providers keep records about our diagnoses, treatments, and test results, patients should do the same. Especially in this era of medical specialization, it is in your own best interest to keep track of what each provider tells you. There are many ways to do so, including through Web sites, with computer memory sticks, or in paper files. The medical record I keep for myself is a three-ring binder with tabbed sections for:

- *Medical reports.* I include copies of pathology reports and discharge instructions. Having these easily available helped not only me but, at times, also my providers. I remember an early-morning procedure that was almost delayed because the specialist didn't have (or couldn't find) a copy of the needed referral. Thanks to my notebook, I had a copy of the needed paperwork.
- *Doctors.* I had so many appointments at different facilities that sometimes I felt like a "secret shopper" of medical matters. To keep track of all these providers, I had a section in my notebook for information about each doctor, including a photo (if available), contact information, and directions to his or her office.

- *Questions.* At home, I could think of lots of questions I wanted to ask my doctors. But when wearing a skimpy hospital johnny, I struggled to remember any of them. To help, I would make a list of all my questions beforehand so that later all I needed to do was write down the answers.
- *Medication lists, healthcare proxies, and other important papers.* Many providers ask similar questions about medications and allergies. I got tired of repeating myself and so made a master list for each office to copy. I also keep my signed healthcare proxy and give a copy to health providers, as requested.
- *Zippered pouch.* I found that a three-hole-punch zippered pouch was a most handy addition to my notebook. I used it as a catch-all for my patient identification cards and doctors' business cards. And when I got tired of fumbling around for a pen for taking notes, I added one to my trusty zippered pouch.

 Providers need to present information about new diagnoses, treatment options, and self-care instructions. Patients need to describe their symptoms, ask questions, and express opinions about treatment and care. And both need to listen closely, respond thoughtfully, and remember clearly what each other just said.

CITATIONS

Osborne H. 2005. In other words . . . From Another Point of View . . . A Patient's Perspective About Health Communication. *On Call.* Available at http://www .healthliteracy.com/patient-perspective. Accessed April 20, 2011.

Osborne H. 2006. In Other Words . . . Communicating When Naked: My Perspective as a Patient. *On Call.* Available at http://www.healthliteracy.com/communicating-when-naked. Accessed April 20, 2011.

SOURCES TO LEARN MORE

Chen PW. 2009, April 2. Do You Know What Your Doctor Is Talking About? *New York Times.* Available at http://www.nytimes.com/2009/04/02/health/02chen.html. Accessed April 16, 2011.

DeMarco RF, Picard C, Agretelis J. 2004. Nurse Experiences as Cancer Survivors: Part I—Personal. *Oncology Nursing Forum.* 31(3):523–530.

Osborne H. 2007. In Other Words . . . When Providers Are Patients. *On Call.* Available at http://www.healthliteracy.com/providers-as-patients. Accessed April 20, 2011.

Osborne H. 2009. The More You Know: How Much Is Enough When It Comes to Cancer Information? *CureToday.com*. Available at http://www.curetoday .com/index.cfm/fuseaction/article.show/id/2/article_id/1360 Accessed April 16, 2011.

Picard C, Agretelis J, DeMarco RF. 2004. Nurse Experiences as Cancer Survivors: Part II—Professional. *Oncology Nursing Forum*. 31(3):537–542.

Towle A. 2006. Where's the Patient's Voice in Health Professional Education? *Nurse Education in Practice*. 6(5):300–302.

U.S. Department of Health and Human Services, National Institutes of Health, National Cancer Institute. 2004. *Surgery Choices for Women with Early Stage Breast Cancer*. NIH Publication No. 04-5515. [Currently not available, pending revision]

Confirming Understanding: Feedback from Interviews, Focus Groups, and Usability Testing

STARTING POINTS

Regardless of the material you are creating (such as printed documents or Web sites), it is well worthwhile to confirm understanding by asking for feedback from people who represent the intended audience. Whether you get this feedback by interviewing people one-on-one, meeting with them in focus groups, or observing them during usability tests, audience feedback is helpful throughout the writing process.

When writing patient educational booklets, for example, you can use feedback at the beginning of projects to determine topics to include. As you write, you can use feedback to assess how clearly you communicate key points. And when the project is complete, readers can provide feedback about what to do differently in the next edition.

As valuable as feedback is, it is an often overlooked and omitted step. In part, this may be because interviews, focus groups, and usability testing take time and cost money. It may also be that writers (or committees) are under deadline to get newly written documents into use. And sometimes feedback doesn't happen because writers feel they already know the reader's perspective. But this is seldom the case. Writers are usually so familiar with the content that they cannot objectively judge whether words and concepts make sense to others.

Stories from Practice: Benefits of Asking for Feedback

Constanza Villalba, PhD, is a proponent of reader feedback. As the Associate Editor of patient information for the UpToDate Web site, Villalba oversaw the process of rewriting patient information at a more basic level. She asked adult basic education students, non-medical professionals, and doctors or other subject-matter experts for their feedback.

Villalba said that doing so was extremely helpful. Beyond learning more about the documents themselves, she said that this process helped refute any "pushback" from those who questioned whether revised materials were now too simple. The feedback process "gave me backup and backbone," says Villalba.

Source: Villalba (2010).

STRATEGIES, IDEAS, AND SUGGESTIONS

Here are some strategies to put into practice (Osborne 2005, 2010):

Know your intended audience. At the start of new projects, find out about the learning abilities, information needs, language, and culture of your intended audience. Beyond looking at demographics, meet with several potential readers and ask what types of information they require. For example, in addition to self-care instructions, readers may be interested in how much a procedure costs or how often they will need follow-up appointments.

Ask for opinions. When you ask people to review materials, make it clear that you are testing the material and not their reading or comprehension skills. Make sure you ask questions in ways that help people feel comfortable expressing opinions. Begin by asking, "Will you help me?" Then let people know how you will use their feedback, and offer to show them updated versions.

Budget both time and money. Admittedly, reader feedback usually takes time and costs money. But the need for these resources should not be considered a "deal breaker." Think creatively about ways to get feedback as part of your regular business. For example, instead of making appointments for interviews, you could ask patients for opinions while they sit in the clinic's waiting room.

Get feedback throughout the process. Feedback is beneficial at all stages of the writing process. After you complete a first draft and are reasonably confident that your material is clear and easy to read, ask intended readers for their feedback. Once you make revisions based on their feedback, ask again to make sure you didn't introduce new problems. Continue this process until your readers confirm that they truly understand.

Conduct interviews. Interviewing one person at a time is a flexible and effective way to get feedback. This technique can be particularly useful when asking for opinions from people who fear embarrassment (perhaps due to limited literacy), are unaccustomed to giving opinions in front of others, or lack the fluency needed to speak up. Here are some ways:

- Plan questions ahead of time. Frame questions as open-ended queries, such as "What do you like about the pictures in this booklet?" rather than yes/no choices, like "Does this booklet look good to you?"
- Observe how people engage with your material. For example, notice whether people smile when looking at the illustrations or seem confused by the charts and graphs.
- Encourage interviewees to "think aloud" and to talk about their reactions as they read the entire document.

Use focus groups. Focus groups and other forms of consumer testing of written materials are other effective ways of getting feedback. Generally, groups have six to eight people who represent the audience in terms of age, literacy, language, culture, and familiarity with the subject matter. Most groups are co-led by a trained facilitator who asks questions and a recorder who takes notes. You might want to test your material with more than one focus group. This way, you can compare responses from different groups. For example, you could test a booklet about hospital services with a group of people who were hospitalized on an emergency basis and those who had planned admissions.

Conduct usability testing. You can learn how user-friendly your document or Web site is through usability testing—controlled settings or labs in which you observe people using your materials. Such studies involve asking people to complete specific tasks, such as navigating around a Web site. As the tester, you observe which aspects of tasks are easy, or hard, for people to do. And then use these observations to determine which changes to make.

 You can use feedback at the beginning of the project to determine which topics to include. As you write, you can use feedback to assess how clearly you are communicating key messages. And when the project is complete, readers can provide feedback about what to change in the next revision.

CITATIONS

Osborne H. 2005. In Other Words . . . Listening to Your Audience . . . How to Get Reader Feedback. *On Call*. Available at http://www.healthliteracy.com/ reader-feedback. Accessed April 20, 2011.

Osborne H (host). 2010, March 23. Creating Usable, Useful Health Websites for Readers at All Levels [audio podcast]. *Health Literacy Out Loud*, no. 34. Available at http://www.healthliteracy.com/hlol-websites-for-all-readers. Accessed April 20, 2011.

Villalba C. 2010. Personal communication.

SOURCES TO LEARN MORE

Brugge D, Edgar T, George K, Heung J, Laws MB. 2009. Beyond Literacy and Numeracy in Patient Provider Communication: Focus Groups Suggest Roles for Empowerment, Provider Attitude and Language. *BMC Public Health*. 9:354. Available at http://www.biomedcentral.com/1471-2458/9/354. Accessed June 2, 2011.

Krueger RA, Casey MA. 2000. *Focus Groups: A Practical Guide for Applied Research*, 3rd ed. Thousand Oaks, CA: Sage.

Office of Disease Prevention and Health Promotion (ODPHP), National Health Information Center. 2011. *Quick Guide to Healthy Living*. Available at http:// www.healthfinder.gov/prevention. Accessed January 8, 2011.

Office of Disease Prevention and Health Promotion, U.S. Department of Health and Human Services. 2009, October 20. Health Literacy Online: Building an Easy-to-Use Health Information Web Site. *Health Literacy Month*. Available at http://www .healthliteracy.com/hlmonth-building-website. Accessed April 16, 2011.

Osborne H. 2001. In Other Words . . . Can They Understand? Testing Patient Education Materials with Intended Readers. *On Call*. Available at http://www .healthliteracy.com/testing-materials-with-readers. Accessed April 20, 2011.

Osborne H. 2005. In Other Words . . . What Makes Web Sites Patient-Friendly? *On Call*. Available at http://www.healthliteracy.com/patient-friendly-websites. Accessed April 20, 2011.

Osborne H (host). 2009, August 13. Communicating Clearly on the Web [audio podcast]. *Health Literacy Out Loud*, no. 19. Available at http://www.healthliteracy .com/hlol-web. Accessed April 20, 2011.

Osborne H (host). 2010. August 10. Press Ganey's CEO Talks About Analyzing Sentiments to Improve Healthcare Quality [audio podcast]. *Health Literacy Out Loud*, no. 43. Available at http://healthliteracy.com/hlol-sentiment-analysis. Accessed April 20, 2011.

Quesenbery W, Brooks K. 2010. *Storytelling for User Experience: Crafting Stories for Better Design*. Brooklyn, NY: Rosenfeld Media.

Redish J. 2007. *Letting Go of the Words: Writing Web Content That Works*. San Francisco, CA: Morgan Kaufmann.

Sudman S, Bradburn NM. 1982. *Asking Questions: A Practical Guide to Questionnaire Design*. San Francisco: Jossey-Bass.

UpToDate, Inc., www.uptodate.com

Usability.gov: Your Guide for Developing Usable and Useful Web Sites. U.S. Department of Health and Human Services, www.usability.gov/templates/index.html.

U.S. Department of Health and Human Services, Centers for Medicare and Medicaid Services, by Jeanne McGee of McGee & Evers Consulting. 2010. *Toolkit for Making Written Material Clear and Effective*. Available at http://www.cms.gov/WrittenMaterialsToolkit/. Accessed January 8, 2011.

Confirming Understanding: Teach-Back Technique

STARTING POINTS

The teach-back technique (also known as the "interactive communication loop") is a way to assess and confirm whether patients truly understand the provider's spoken words.

Providers can use this technique to assess a patient's recall and comprehension of important concepts just discussed. If the patient does not understand a concept correctly or completely, then the provider restates or tailors the message to make it more accessible. The provider again assesses the patient's comprehension and continues this process until it is clear that the patient understands.

STRATEGIES, IDEAS, AND SUGGESTIONS

Here are some helpful strategies (Osborne 2003):

Set a tone of partnership. Patients need to feel safe admitting that they don't understand. Schillinger invites patients to be partners, beginning with a statement like, "I want to make sure that you and I are on the same page." He then asks open-ended questions about new concepts, such as, "Now that we've talked about adding fiber to your diet, what will you look for the next time you buy cereal?" If the patient seems confused or doesn't know the answer, Schillinger will offer an empathic statement such as, "Many people have trouble figuring out which cereals are high in fiber."

Stories from Practice: A Time-Efficient and Cost-Effective Technique to Confirm Understanding

Dean Schillinger, MD, is a professor of medicine at the University of California, San Francisco, and San Francisco General Hospital. In his research about healthcare communication, Schillinger found that, at best, patients recall and comprehend only about half of the information delivered in a clinical encounter. "It's a flip of a coin that what you say (and how you say it) has sunk in," he says. Schillinger routinely uses the interactive communication loop to determine whether patients truly understand key messages.

Schillinger knows that some providers are reluctant to open the communication loop, fearing it will take too much time. But he says he has found the technique is both time-efficient and time-effective. When providers know what patients understand and accept, they can specifically focus on the most important aspects of the message. "Used well and used often," says Schillinger, "the communication loop is an efficient way to get to where you need to be."

Source: Osborne (2003).

The one question that Schillinger does not use to assess understanding is, "Do you understand?" He says that most patients, whether or not they understand, simply respond by nodding and smiling. Rather, he suggests placing the onus of misunderstanding on the clinician or educator by asking, "I just want to make sure I explained things well. When you go home and your husband asks what the doctor suggested about your medication, what will you tell him?"

Tailor your message to be more consistent with what the patient says. Just like with clothes, tailoring means altering the message to fit each person's frame of understanding. For example, the statement "exercise more" is an untailored message. To tailor this message, use an example familiar to each patient. When talking about exercise with someone who likes to swim, you might say, "Instead of swimming just once a week like you have been doing, try to swim three times a week for at least a half an hour."

Consider why the message is not understood. Even when you believe you have given an adequate explanation, patients still may not understand. When this happens, consider if there are other factors such as learning disabilities, hearing loss, cognitive impairments, depression, limited literacy or language skills, or cultural differences that are getting in the way. If so, look for ways to overcome these factors, such as by bringing in an interpreter, inviting a family member to join the conversation, or making an appointment focused solely on teaching.

Stories from Practice: Actively Listen for What Patients Do Not Say

Elyse Barbell is executive director of the Literacy Assistance Center in New York City. While she's a big believer in the importance of using teach-back, Barbell recommends the additional step of actively listening for what patients do not say. She shares strategies for active listening:

- Pay attention not just to peoples' words but also their body language, eye contact, and tone of voice.
- Don't be satisfied when a patient's teach-back is just "pretty good." Instead, listen for what the patient didn't say. What was left out can reflect gaps in understanding.
- Respond specifically to patients' teach-back. Barbell says that clinicians owe patients at least one more sentence rather than simply ending with "Okay, thank you."
- Reinforce lessons that patients learned well. For instance, you can say, "You got that just right and really understand that one of the most important things you can do is . . . "
- Teach key content again when you notice discrepancies. For instance, make a statement such as, "You said that really well, but what I didn't hear was . . . . That's really important to do, and I want to make sure you know how."
- Supplement teaching with good take-home (written) instructions. Choose materials that have informative illustrations, simply stated step-by-step instructions, and vocabulary matching your spoken word.
- Continue teaching and asking for teach-back until you are assured that patients fully understand. "If patients cannot follow how to do a task with you sitting there, there is zero chance they will do it at home," says Barbell.

Source: Osborne (2008).

The teach-back technique (also known as the "interactive communication loop") is a way to assess and confirm whether patients truly understand the provider's spoken words.

CITATIONS

Osborne H. 2003. In Other Words . . . Opening the Interactive Communication Loop."
On Call. Available at http://www.healthliteracy.com/interactive-communication-loop. Accessed April 20, 2011.

Osborne H. 2008. In Other Words . . . Actively Listening for What Patients Do Not Say. *On Call.* Available at http://www.healthliteracy.com/active-listening Accessed April 20, 2011.

SOURCES TO LEARN MORE

Kemp EC, Floyd MR, McCord-Duncan E, Lang F. 2008. Patients Prefer the Method of "Tell Back-Collaborative Inquiry" to Assess Understanding of Medical Information. *Journal of the American Board of Family Medicine.* 21(1):24–30.

Osborne H (host). 2009, May 5. Terry Davis Talks About "Baby Steps" (Action Planning) [audio podcast]. *Health Literacy Out Loud,* no. 16. Available at http://www.healthliteracy.com/hlol-action-planning. Accessed January 8, 2011.

Schillinger D, Piette J, Grumbach K, Wang F, Wilson C, Daher C, et al. 2003. Closing the Loop: Physician Communication with Diabetic Patients Who Have Low Health Literacy. *Archives of Internal Medicine.* 163(1):83–90.

Decision Aids and Shared Decision-Making

STARTING POINTS

In the United States today, patients are often asked by their doctors to participate in making decisions about important aspects of treatment and care. For instance, this might be to choose between two surgery options, or decide whether to begin treatment now or wait to see if symptoms get worse.

In this process of "shared decision-making," the doctor or other healthcare provider presents the patient with options (treatment choices, including medical interventions or active surveillance), outcomes (what is likely to happen), probabilities (chances that these outcomes will occur), and uncertainties (what is unknown or not determined). The patient, in turn, shares his or her values and concerns about the benefits and harms of treatment alternatives. Together, providers and patients plan a course of action.

Today, patients are increasingly activated and engaged in all aspects of treatment and care. While the examples below are about breast cancer, shared decision-making is a factor for all diagnoses and conditions.

STRATEGIES, IDEAS, AND SUGGESTIONS

Here are some suggestions you might find useful (Osborne 2004; Finn 2011):

Find out how much patients want to be involved in decision-making. While many patients want to be actively involved in decision-making, others may look more to doctors, family members, or trusted advisers for guidance.

Stories from Practice: A Patient's Experience of Decision-Making

Kathryn Sabadosa is a health professional. She is also a patient who was diagnosed with breast cancer. Sabadosa clearly recalls feeling like her world fell apart when the pathologist called to say that she had cancer. Soon thereafter, a social worker contacted Sabadosa to introduce the concept of shared decision-making and offer guidance throughout this process.

Sabadosa's social worker lent her some learning resources ("decision aids") that included a video and companion booklet about surgery choices. These defined important words, explained possible risks, and described what to expect from each type of surgery. Most important, the video had stories from several women who each spoke in an unbiased way about the treatment choice she had made.

Sabadosa offers advice to others making important medical decisions:

- Take time to gather information and think about all the choices before you make a decision.
- Be comfortable with the professionals providing your care. For instance, Sabadosa wanted a doctor who would listen, not just tell her what to do.
- Make clear how much you want to be involved in decisions. This includes not allowing even trusted family members to override your decision. As Sabadosa says, "It's your body. You have to live with the outcome and look in the mirror each day."

Source: Sabadosa (2010).

Assess each patient's willingness to participate in the decision-making process. As needed and if possible, refer patients to trained "decision support specialists," such as a nurse, social worker, or behavioral health counselor.

Acknowledge the importance of feelings and values. Decisions that patients make may be influenced as much by feelings and values as they are by facts. For example, some patients are uncomfortable with uncertainty and opt for treatment that has the most assured outcomes. Help patients sort through and clarify their feelings throughout the decision-making process.

Stories from Practice: Create a System That Offers Decision-Making Support

---

If your practice routinely presents patients with treatment options, you might want to create a system that offers decision-making support. Jeff Belkora, PhD, runs the Decision Services program at the University of California–San Francisco Medical Center's Carol Franc Buck Breast Care Center.

This service is designed to help women newly diagnosed with breast cancer reflect critically on decisions they are about to make. Belkora says that this service helps women "slow down and appreciate the subtleties of other approaches" rather than following their initial "fight, flight, or freeze reactions."

Between the time of diagnosis and first appointment with a breast cancer specialist, a trained decision-support counselor contacts each patient. The counselor not only provides teaching resources and decision aids but also offers to accompany the patient to her appointments. Belkora says that decision-making services such as these are so successful that there are plans to create more.

Source: Osborne (2010, November 30).

Use decision aids and other teaching tools to present information in understandable ways. As defined on the Web site of the Ottawa Hospital Research Institute (OHRI), "Patient decision aids are tools that help people become involved in decision making by providing information about the options and outcomes and by clarifying personal values. They are designed to complement, rather than replace, counseling from a health practitioner." Decision aids include personal assessments, videos, booklets, and other informative or individualized resources.

Here are other strategies for communicating information needed to make decisions:

- **Metaphors.** These are used to compare new concepts to those that are more familiar. For instance, when presenting risks, in addition to giving data you might also say, "The chance that [x] will happen is about the same as catching a baseball when sitting in the bleachers at Fenway Park." (Read more in the "Metaphors, Similes, and Analogies" chapter, starting on page 139.)

- **Numbers.** When discussing data, confirm that the patient is comfortable with and savvy about using numbers. You can supplement data with pictures or comparisons to known quantities. You can also use gestures, such as holding one hand up to indicate high, and the other down, conveying low. (Read more in "Numeracy" chapter, starting on page 143.)
- **Research data.** When presenting data from clinical trials and research studies, make sure to discuss how to interpret results. This means noting whether the subjects in the study are similar to the patient in terms of age, gender, race, and diagnosis. It also means making sense of ambiguous findings and unanswered questions.

"Shared decision-making" is a process in which the provider presents the patient with options, outcomes, probabilities, and uncertainties. The patient, in turn, shares his or her values and concerns about the benefits and harms of treatment alternatives. Together, providers and patients plan a course of action.

CITATIONS

Finn C. 2011. Personal communication.

Osborne H. 2004. In Other Words . . . Helping Patients Make Difficult Decisions. *On Call.* Available at http://www.healthliteracy.com/difficult-decisions. Accessed April 20, 2011.

Osborne H (host). 2010, November 30. Decision Support for Patients Making Life-Changing Choices [audio podcast]. *Health Literacy Out Loud,* no. 49. Available at http://www.healthliteracy.com/hlol-decision-support. Accessed January 8, 2011.

Ottawa Health Research Institute. n.d. *Ottawa Personal Decision Guide.* Available at decisionaid.ohri.ca/decguide.html. Accessed January 10, 2011.

Sabadosa K. 2010. Telephone interview.

SOURCES TO LEARN MORE

Dartmouth-Hitchcock Medical Center, Center for Shared Decision Making, www.hitchcock.org/dept/csdm

Foundation for Informed Medical Decision Making, www.informedmedicaldecisions.org

Health Dialog, www.healthdialog.com

Katz SJ, Lantz PM, Janz NK, Fagerlin A, Schwartz K, Liu L, et al. Patient Involvement in Surgery Treatment Decisions for Breast Cancer. *Journal of Clinical Oncology.* 23(24):5526–5533.

Lantz PM, Janz NK, Fagerlin A, Schwartz K, Liu L, Lakhani I, et al. 2005. Satisfaction with Surgery Outcomes and the Decision Process in a Population-Based Sample of Women with Breast Cancer. *Health Services Research.* 40(3):745–768.

UCSF Medical Center. 2009. *The Carol Franc Buck Breast Care Center: Decision Services.* Available at http://decisionservices.ucsf.edu. Accessed April 16, 2011.

Document Design

Starting Points

Printed and Web materials not only need to be written clearly and simply, they also should be designed in ways that readers find inviting and appealing. "Information design" refers to the art of doing just that, combining words and images to encourage readers to start, and keep, reading.

Strategies, Ideas, and Suggestions

Consider the following elements when designing your documents (Osborne 2009, December 7):

- **Use headings and subheads.** Headings identify key sections, while subheads mark topics within. Both make it easier for readers to find the information that they want and need. For instance, in this chapter there is the heading, "Document Design." Then there are several subheads, "Strategies, Ideas, and Suggestions," "Citations," and "Sources to Learn More." As you can see, these are differentiated from the rest of the text using design elements including FONT, size, *italics*, and **bold**.
- **Choose an appropriate font type.** Which font should you use? A "serif font" with extra ascenders and descenders, like Times New Roman? Or a "sans serif" or "block" font like Arial? Schriver (1997) answered this age-old question, "If you're designing on paper, it's usually a good

Stories from Practice: Readers' Emotional Response to Text and Graphics

Karen Schriver, PhD, is an expert on information design and author of *Dynamics in Document Design: Creating Texts for Readers*. In a *Health Literacy Out Loud* podcast, she highlighted the importance of document design. "Readers can feel respected and valued when two things happen. One, when they understand the text; when they actually 'get' whatever is being said via words and graphics. The second is when they feel as though the text itself responds to them emotionally."

"When people look at a text that is confusing, they don't feel respected because they feel as though they're not being talked to, just being talked at. An example is a pamphlet with difficult words, complicated sentences, or paragraphs that go on and on and on. Good information design considers the reader's likely emotional response to text and graphics. We know from years of research that reading isn't just an intellectual cognitive activity. It's an emotional activity, as well," says Schriver.

Source: Osborne (2009, December 7).

idea to present your body text using a serif font. When designing for the Web, generally speaking it's a good idea to go with sans-serif fonts because they are cleaner and much easier to see with light projecting behind them."

- **Use an appropriate font size.** Make it a habit to use at least 12-point type size. This is large enough for most readers to see. When writing for older adults or those with vision problems, you might want to "bump up" to at least 14-point font size. The standard for large print is 16- to 18-point font. (Read more in "Know Your Audience: Vision Problems," starting on page 127.)

- **Use both upper- and lower-case letters.** Perhaps you've heard not to use all capital letters because this looks like shouting. Honestly, I haven't a clue whether or not this is true. But there is at least one compelling reason to combine upper- and lower-case letters: lower-case letters offer important visual clues with their varying heights.

Let's say I'm writing about my trip to Africa. Without looking closely, can you recognize these words?

- **ELEPHANTS AND GIRAFFES.** This can be hard to see as the same-sized lettering gives it the overall shape of a rectangle.
- **elephants and giraffes.** When the letters "p" and "g" descend (go down), and "l," "h," "t," and "f" ascend (go up), there are visual cues as to the meaning of these words. Add the fact that you already know the context for these words (that I'm writing about my trip to Africa), and you're even more likely to figure out these words.

- **Justify the left margin.** Line up (justify) your text on the left so that each line starts at the same place. But do not justify on the right or center the text, as either of these may result in odd-sized spacing.
- **Use short, bulleted lists.** As you can see from the design of this book, I'm a fan of bulleted lists. But I do urge some restraint. Do not over-whelm readers with too many lists, or too many items within each list. Instead try to limit bulleted lists to just 6–8 items. If you need to include more items than that, divide the list into subgroups.

For example, instead of listing 15 types of fruit in one long list, divide it into shorter bulleted lists. Here is an example:

Citrus fruit:
- Grapefruit
- Lemons
- Limes
- Oranges
- Tangerines

Melons:
- Cantaloupe
- Casaba
- Honeydew
- Muskmelon
- Watermelon

Tropical fruit:
- Banana
- Mango
- Papya
- Pineapple
- Pomegranate

- **Maintain "adequate" white space.** But what is adequate? My sassy answer is that you know it when you see it. A more analytic response is that adequate white space means having about a 50/50 mix between printed and unprinted areas on each page.
- **Consider contrast.** Schriver is a strong proponent of using contrast in written documents. This includes having headings that are bolder than the rest of the text, pictures that range in size from large to small, and colors that distinguish certain parts of the page. "Readers will scan the text for those things that jump out at them," says Schriver. "One key principle of information design is to capitalize on that natural attraction to contrast and build it into your document," she says (Osborne 2009).
- **Remember subjectivity and opinion.** Jeanne McGee, PhD, is author of the *Toolkit for Making Material Clear and Effective*. She provides detailed instruction about designing written health materials. Beyond guidelines about what to do and why, McGee offers some caution. "Design is an art, not a science, with lots of room for subjective judgment and differences in taste." She adds that applying design guidelines to your own materials is both an "art and an adventure" (U.S. Department of Health and Human Services, *Toolkit*, Ch. 2, p. 11).

 Information design refers to the art of combining words and images to encourage readers to start, and keep, reading.

Citations

Osborne H (host). December 7, 2009. Using Design to Get Readers to Read and Keep Reading [audio podcast]. *Health Literacy Out Loud,* no. 29. Available at http://www.healthliteracy.com/hlol-design-principles. Accessed January 10, 2011.

Schriver KA. 1997. *Dynamics in Document Design: Creating Texts for Readers.* New York: John Wiley & Sons.

U.S. Department of Health and Human Services, Centers for Medicare and Medicaid Services, by Jeanne McGee of McGee & Evers Consulting. 2010. Guidelines for Overall Design and Page Layout. *Toolkit for Making Written Material Clear and Effective.* Available at http://www.cms.gov/WrittenMaterialsToolkit/07_ToolkitPart05.asp. Accessed January 8, 2011.

Sources to Learn More

Emerson J. 2008. *Visualising Information for Advocacy.* Tactical Technology Collective. Available at http://www.tacticaltech.org/visualisingadvocacy. Accessed January 10, 2011.

Schriver KA. n.d. *Info Design: Understanding by Design* [blog]. Available at http://www .informationdesign.org/. Accessed January 10, 2011.

Wheildon C. 1995. *Type and Layout: How Typography and Design Can Get Your Message Across—or Get in the Way.* Berkeley, CA: Strathmoor.

Williams R. 1994. *The Non-Designer's Design Book: Design and Typographic Principles for the Visual Novice.* Berkeley, CA: Pearson Education.

Environment of Care: Entrances, Questions, Signs, and Feng Shui

STARTING POINTS

Have you ever considered what it feels like to be a new patient or visitor at your hospital or clinic? Not just how it feels to be sick or scared, but what it is like to wend your way around someplace new? And once you are where you need to be, does the space feel welcoming and conducive to talking about health? It is not just written materials and oral communication that impacts health literacy. Environment of care matters, too.

STRATEGIES, IDEAS, AND SUGGESTIONS

Many people, from many perspectives, are adding to our knowledge about the environment of care. The suggestions below are based on interviews and conversations with experts in health literacy, architecture, and accessibility—Rima Rudd (Osborne 2001), Todd Hansen (2009), and Valerie Fletcher (Osborne 2010, October 5).

Consider the outside entrance. Hospitals and clinics are busy places, with people coming in and out all sorts of doors. Consider how your patients and visitors determine which one to use. Sometimes a sign such as "Ambulatory Entrance" adds to confusion, as patients might assume this entrance is for ambulances, not patients. Instead, use simpler and more familiar wording, such as "Patient Entrance."

Stories from Practice: What Zoos Can Teach Us About Navigation

Oddly enough, health literacy came to mind when I visited the elephant house at the Chicago Zoological Society's Brookfield Zoo. I had a question about the exhibit and then suddenly noticed the answer on a sign right in front of me. It was so well placed it made me wonder what we in health care might learn from zoos.

To find out, I contacted Jo-Elle E. H. Mogerman, PhD, vice president of planning and community relations for the Chicago Zoological Society, and Andre Copeland, the Society's public programs manager. They explained the role of design, wording, and placement of signs in helping zoo visitors get where they want to go and learn while they're getting there.

Mogerman and Copeland also spoke of Maslow's hierarchy of needs, how they keep in mind what is most important to a visitor at any particular point. For instance, when people enter the Brookfield Zoo, two of the first things they want to know are where the bathrooms are and where they can get something to eat. In their opinion as well as mine, considering what is foremost to patients and families can be equally effective in healthcare settings.

Source: Osborne (2007).

Anticipate first-visit questions. Many people have lots of questions when first visiting a facility. These include: Do I need to register or check in? What time are visiting hours? Where do I go for my test or procedure? Here are some ways to help patients learn the answers:

- Have a designated "Information Desk" in the lobby. Staff might include employees or volunteers who not only know their way around the facility but also are friendly and happy to help.
- Provide accurate, readable, and up-to-date facility maps. Make sure that the font size is sufficiently large for people to see. Confirm that departments have not moved since the last time the map was published. Use wording that matches what people know and are looking for, such as "Mammogram" instead of "Women's Health." And even when maps meet all these criteria, know that there will always be people who cannot, or prefer not to, use maps.

- Consider having information kiosks or other types of technology. Just like everywhere else in our lives, technology is increasingly being looked to as a way to help people navigate new places. While today you might have touch-screen kiosks to answer common questions, there seem to be limitless options for what technology will come up with tomorrow.

Provide appropriate signage. Written and picture-based signs are designed to help people get from place to place. But signs are not always easy to understand or follow. Here are some ways to help:

- **Consider word choice.** Be consistent in the words you use, such as always using the term "dining room" or "cafeteria." Then use this same wording in the sign at the doorway, on facility maps, and in verbal directions.
- **Consider word order.** Many health facilities have patient areas and meeting rooms named for generous donors. But when it comes to signage, putting the donor's name at the top can be confusing. It tends to be easier for newcomers to read signs with a descriptive term at the top, such as "X-Ray," and the benefactor's name below.
- **Use appropriate symbols**. Patients and families today speak a wide variety of languages, come from many different countries, and vary widely in their learning abilities. To help people more easily find their way, consider using pictograms or images along with simple words. Hablamos Juntos, an organization dedicated to language policy and practice in health care, has developed and tested 28 universal healthcare symbols. These include signage for ambulance entrances, cardiology departments, and waiting area. You can download a poster of these symbols at: http://www.hablamosjuntos.org/signage/PDF/SignagePoster(8x11).pdf.

Conduct tours and audits. One of the best ways to find out if your environment of care is easy to navigate is to accompany a newcomer making his or her way around the facility for the very first time. While you don't know for sure that what works for one person will necessarily work for another, informal tours like these can help raise awareness of potential navigation problems. There also is a growing body of resources to audit the healthcare environment in more formalized ways. Resources include:

- Jacobson KL, Gazmararian JA, Kripalani S, McMorris KJ, Blake SC, Brach. 2007. *Is Our Pharmacy Meeting Patients' Needs? A Pharmacy*

Health Literacy Assessment Tool User's Guide. AHRQ publication No. 07-0051. Rockville, MD: Agency for Healthcare Research and Quality. Available at http://www.ahrq.gov/qual/pharmlit/. Accessed January 14, 2011.

- National Adult Literacy Agency (NALA). 2009. *Literacy Audit for Healthcare Settings*. Dublin, Ireland. Available at http://www .healthpromotion.ie/uploads/docs/HSE_NALA_Health_Audit.pdf Accessed January 14, 2011.
- Rudd RE. 2010. *The Health Literacy Environment Activity Packet: First Impressions and Walking Interview* [online tools]. Health Literacy Studies. Available at http://www.hsph.harvard.edu/healthliteracy/resources/ Accessed January 14, 2011.

Incorporate Feng Shui. Patients and providers often discuss intimate health care matters such as life, death, and bodily functions. These very personal and often emotional conversations can be even more difficult when taking place in environments that feel cold and impersonal. Based on an ancient Chinese art, Feng Shui is a way to help create an environment conducive to talking about health. Linda Varone, RN, of Nuturing Spaces Consulting, advises considering the following (Osborne 2001, May).

- **Color.** Medical settings generally have little color, with mostly beige or light pastel walls. Clinicians, too, usually dress in white or light-colored uniforms and jackets. You can add a dose of color and visual interest by using wallpaper borders or decorative room accents like pillows or pictures. And, if your dress code permits, you may also want to wear a colorful pin or scarf on your lab coat or uniform.
- **Sound.** There are many sounds you can't control in healthcare settings, such as overhead announcements, hallway conversations, and equipment being wheeled from one room to another. To counter these, consider playing soothing background music to filter out intrusive sounds.
- **Living things.** People often feel more at ease when they are around living things like plants and animals. While there may be institutional restrictions on bringing in live plants or other living things, consider at least having a silk plant or small stuffed animal.
- **Movement.** Often, little happens in corners. To create a sense of movement and add energy to these quiet spaces, think about adding a mobile, table-top water fountain, or pleasant-sounding wind chime.

- **Texture.** Healthcare settings have a distinctive institutional feel to them, with many hard or cold surfaces like concrete walls and stainless steel furniture. To counteract these, you can introduce a soft throw pillow or fabric table cover.
- **Furniture.** You can create settings that feel private and intimate even when there is built-in furniture and other fixtures you cannot change. You may, for example, use a moveable bookcase to create a sense of privacy. You can also position chairs and beds so that people can see out of doorways and are not surprised when someone enters the room.
- **Artwork.** Personalize spaces by adding calming photographs or artwork. Choose items appropriate to the patients you are treating, such as pictures of older adults for a geriatric clinic. Since people's tastes differ, have a variety of artwork so most everyone finds something to help them feel more at ease.
- **Clutter.** Providers often have books, paperwork, and numerous health-related items scattered about. It can feel cluttered when these objects look messy or not cared for. Like all forms of communication, simplicity helps. Periodically clean out what you display (and also what you store) to give your space a feeling of openness and simplicity.

 It is not just written materials and oral communication that impacts health literacy. Environment of care matters, too.

Citations

Hansen T. 2009. Meeting of the Boston Society of Architects Committee on Healthcare Facilities. Boston, MA.

Osborne H. 2001, May. In Other Words . . . Using Feng Shui to Improve Healthcare Communication. *On Call.* 4(5):46–47. Available at http://www.healthliteracy.com/feng-shui-in-healthcare. Accessed January 13, 2011.

Osborne H. 2001, October. In Other Words . . . Tools to Help Patients Navigate Their Way Around Hospitals. *On Call.* Available at http://www.healthliteracy.com/helping-patients-navigate. Accessed January 13, 2011.

Osborne H. 2007, May 29. In Other Words . . . What Healthcare Settings Can Learn from Zoos About Signage and Wayfinding. *On Call.* Available at http://www.healthliteracy.com/learning-from-zoos-about signage/. Accessed January 13, 2011.

Osborne H (host). 2010, October 5. Universal Design and Health Communication [audio podcast]. *Health Literacy Out Loud,* no. 46. Available at http://www.healthliteracy.com/hlol-universal-design. Accessed January 13, 2011.

Sources to Learn More

Chin RD. 1998. *Feng Shui Revealed*. New York: Clarkson Potter.

Hablamos Juntos, Language Policy and Practice in Health Care, http://hablamosjuntos.org/. Includes *Signs That Work: Universal Symbols for Healthcare*.

Linn D. 1999. *Feng Shui for the Soul: How to Create a Harmonious Environment That Will Nurture and Sustain You*. Carlsbad, CA: Hay House.

Rudd RE, Anderson JE. 2006. *The Health Literacy Environment of Hospitals and Health Centers—Partners for Action: Making Your Healthcare Facility Literacy-Friendly*. National Center for the Study of Adult Learning and Literacy, and Health and Adult Literacy and Learning Initiative, Harvard School of Public Health. Available at http://www.hsph.harvard.edu/healthliteracy/resources/index.html. Accessed January 13, 2011.

Rudd RE, Rezulli D, Perreira A, Daltroy LD. 2004. The Patient Health Experience. In Schwartzberg JG, VanGeest JB, Want CC, Gazmararian JA, Parker RM, Roter DL, et al. (eds.). *Understanding Health Literacy: Implications for Medicine and Public Health*. Chicago: AMA Press; 69–84.

Ethics of Simplicity

STARTING POINTS

In many ways, plain-language writers act as translators of scientific and medical information—communicating complicated, rapidly changing, numbers-based, often ambiguous health information in a manner that is sufficiently clear and simple for "average" readers to understand.

This task is much more difficult than simply replacing multisyllabic terms with one- and two-syllable words. As I know from many years as a plain-language writer, there are often dilemmas to resolve and issues to consider. I've long referred to these as the "ethics of simplicity."

STRATEGIES, IDEAS, AND SUGGESTIONS

Here are some ideas to consider (Osborne 2004):

Be clear about why you are writing this document. A good way to identify project goals is by asking yourself what readers should know, do, and feel after reading this document. Use these goals to determine which is essential "need-to-know" information that must be included and what is "nice-to-know" background information that can be deleted.

When writing about diabetes, for example, need-to-know information may be about nutrition and exercise, while nice-to-know information can be about physiology of the digestive process. Of course, some reference to

Stories from Practice: Ethical Dilemmas and Challenges

Andrea Gwosdow, PhD, is president of Gwosdow Associates Science Consultants. She is also a medical-writing colleague. Together, we have led "Ethics of Simplicity" workshops for the American Medical Writers Association. Gwosdow and I polled medical writers about their ethical dilemmas and challenges when writing health materials for consumers.

Ethical dilemmas and challenges include:

- Am I including too much information and overloading readers?
- Am I including too little information and omitting important facts and statistics?
- Is the tone appealing and respectful, or does it sound condescending?
- Are the statistics simple enough for readers to understand, yet complete enough for them to make reasoned choices?
- Are my sources credible and unbiased?
- What is the best way to explain complicated medical concepts when even scientists and physicians disagree?

Gwosdow and I admit that we don't have answers to these and many other ethical challenges and dilemmas. But we do believe that it is important for all medical writers to weigh the implications of such choices throughout the writing process.

physiology can help readers understand why exercise and proper nutrition are recommended.

Create a writing team. This team can help weigh choices and determine which information to include or omit. At a minimum, your writing team should include: (1) subject-matter expert(s), such as scientists or clinicians who verify content accuracy, (2) a plain-language writer who not only knows how to write clearly and simply but also is an unceasing advocate for the reader, and (3) one or more readers who represent your intended audience. Opinions from experts and readers are equally important. As a writer, your job is to present information in ways that satisfy the needs of both.

Use plain language. Using plain language means putting information into context with examples, stories, and metaphors and formatting the document to be inviting and easy to read. Plain language also means using words people already know and defining ones they must learn. Here are some dilemmas and challenges writers often face:

- Sometimes even seemingly "simple" words can cause problems. For example, the word "suggest" can easily be misinterpreted. Even though scientists know that the phrase "study data suggest" refers to preliminary data, lay readers may conclude that the term indicates more certainty than that. You can help by putting words like "may," "might," and "could" into context and clarifying terms that are potentially misunderstood.
- Numbers, especially very large ones, can pose concerns because they are hard for most people to comprehend. When talking about statistics, for example, it's generally easier for people to understand "about 1 out of every 3 people" than "3,289 people out of 10,000." Since people often prefer percentages, you can add in parentheses (33%).
- Carefully designed graphics such as tables or pie charts can also help make statistics clear. One way to make sure tables are easy to read is by having just two or three columns of the most pertinent information. And when appropriate, round numbers out to no more than one decimal figure, such as "26.2" instead of "26.215."

Research your references. Where information comes from is as important as how it is presented. Use the best data available to help readers make wise and informed decisions. This often means doing your own literature search, starting with articles in peer-reviewed journals. Once you are sure that data have been rigorously evaluated, supplement the studies with information found in "gray literature" (non-peer-reviewed materials like magazines, newsletters, and conference proceedings), on Web sites, and from product materials.

Alert readers to possible uncertainty and ambiguity. Another potential concern is the fact that medical information is constantly changing, and even experts may disagree about what is correct. For instance, should people eat a lot of high-fat protein foods or more low-fat grains? Ambiguity needs to be both acknowledged and addressed so your readers are not misled. One way is to preface information by stating that scientists continue to study and learn, letting readers know that what seems correct today may change tomorrow.

Ambiguity needs to be both acknowledged and addressed so your readers are not misled. One way is to state that scientists continue to study and learn, letting readers know that what seems correct today may change tomorrow.

CITATION

Osborne H. 2004. In Other Words . . . The Ethics of Simplicity. *On Call.* Available at http://www.healthliteracy.com/ethics-of-simplicity. Accessed August 1, 2010.

SOURCES TO LEARN MORE

American Medical Writers Association, http://www.amwa.org

Ogden J, Branson R, Bryett A, Campbell A, Febles A, Ferguson I, et al. 2003. What's in a Name? An Experimental Study of Patients' Views of the Impact and Function of a Diagnosis. *Family Practice.* 20(3):248–253.

Osborne H (host). 2011, April 5. Helping Others Understand Health Messages [audio podcast]. Health Literacy Out Loud, no. 56. Available at http://healthliteracy .com/hlol-understand-health-messages. Accessed April 15, 2011.

Forms and Other "Reading-to-Do" Documents

Health care is filled with forms and other "reading-to-do" documents. I am using this term in reference to written materials that require readers to perform word-based tasks such as filling in numbers, rating satisfaction, checking off instructions, and signing consent. To accomplish these tasks, readers not only need to comprehend the text but also locate, recall, and enter information from other parts of the same document, from outside materials, or from memory. This is difficult for many people to do.

According to the 2003 *National Assessment of Adult Literacy (NAAL)*, there are three types of literacy:

- **Prose literacy.** Knowledge and skills needed for searching, comprehending, and using continuous text. Examples include newspapers and brochures.
- **Quantitative literacy**. Knowledge and skills needed for making calculations and using numbers embedded in print. Examples include balancing a checkbook, completing an order form, and determining income or expenses.
- **Document literacy**. Knowledge and skills needed to search, comprehend, and use noncontinuous text in various formats. Examples include maps, tables, and drug labels.

NAAL results show that 34 percent of the adults surveyed tested at a below basic or basic level for document literacy. Most people performing at this level can locate a single piece of information in a short and simple piece of text, but may have trouble with tasks requiring them to locate several pieces of information in moderately complicated text. They can solve simple math problems when the numbers and the operations are provided, but may find it difficult to solve the same problems when they must locate the numbers and the operations in a piece of text (Comings & Kirsch 2004).

Strategies, Ideas, and Suggestions

Here are some strategies you might try (Osborne 2003; 2010):

Know your audience. Know generally, not specifically, about the people who will be using your form. This means knowing demographics, including age, literacy level, and languages spoken. It also means learning whether the audience is likely to have physical or cognitive limitations that might impair their ability to see, comprehend, and remember. Be aware, as well, of your readers' fund of knowledge and make sure they are familiar with the types of information needed to complete the form.

Limit your objectives. When writing forms and other reading-to-do documents, ask people only for the information you need now or will need very soon. For example, don't ask people for their children's ages just because you'll need this data sometime later. Instead, ask only when you truly need to know.

Write in a friendly tone. Let readers know at the beginning of your document why you need certain information. For example, start with, "We take pride in patient care at XYZ Medical Center. Please fill out this short survey and let us know how we are doing." Use a conversational tone throughout, referring to readers as "you" and the organization as "we." Don't get bogged down, however, with too many pleasantries. Sometimes an abundance of "please" and "thank you" statements obscures the form's intent. At the end, thank readers for completing the survey and, as with all written materials, include a way to get more information.

Use consistent wording. Be consistent in your wording and make sure that the labels, questions, and instructions ("given information") on your document exactly match its items and answers ("requested information").

Do not, for example, say "Age Group" in one place and "How old are you?" in another. Instead, you might keep the first heading and then ask, "What is your age?"

Stories from Practice: PIN Can Be Troublesome, Too

One reason that documents are sometimes so difficult is that they assume readers understand acronyms and jargon. But this assumption can be incorrect. I was volunteering as a literacy tutor, working with an Egyptian woman new to English. Since we met at the library and because she had young children, I suggested that for one of our lessons she complete the application to get a library card.

We spent the entire session working on this form, which, until now, I thought was clearly written and easy to complete. But I was caught by surprise at how baffled this woman seemed when asked to write down her PIN. Unfamiliar with this acronym for "personal identification number," this woman wondered why she needed a safety pin to get a library card.

Tasks. Reading-to-do documents ask readers to take some sort of action. Here are some ways to make these tasks easier:

- Show, do not just tell, how to take the needed actions. For example, show an answer that is correctly circled rather than underlined, or a date written as mm/dd/yyyy.
- Suggest that readers circle words they do not know and have staff available to explain what these words mean.
- Ask for concrete information such as name, date, time, or place rather than abstract information such as how/why or cause/effect.
- Be specific in your instructions, such as stating whether to "check one box" or "check all that apply."
- Ask for information in a consistent way. For example, ask people only for yes/no responses and not also to complete fill-in-the-blank statements and rate items on a scale from 1 to 5.
- When asking people to add, subtract, multiple, or divide, line up the numerals in rows and columns rather than writing them as words.

Design. Make sure your documents are easy for readers to see and complete. This means having 12-point font or larger, sufficiently large spaces for people to write their answers, and generous white space so the print doesn't look crowded. But please don't squeeze everything onto one page when two are really needed.

Environment. Help people relax and focus on your document by providing a comfortable environment in which they have sufficient time to read, adequate lighting to see, and help available when needed. Encourage staff to offer assistance to those who ask for, or seem to need, some help. You can do this respectfully by saying, "Many people find these forms hard to fill out. Would you like me to help?"

Test your document. Make sure your documents are not only readable but also usable. Here are some ways:

- Assume the role of the reader and ask yourself, "Is this difficult reading?" and "How complex is the task that readers are being asked to do?"
- Try the form yourself and make sure you can complete it within the given time, in the appropriate space, and with the needed information.
- Then test the form with intended readers. Notice where they have difficulty and ask for suggestions about how to improve. Take readers' feedback seriously as you plan to make needed changes.

 To correctly complete forms, readers not only need to comprehend text but also locate, recall, and enter information from other parts of the same document, from outside materials, and from memory. These tasks are difficult for many people to do.

CITATIONS

Comings J, Kirsch I. 2004. Literacy Skills of U.S. Adults. In Schwartzberg JG, Vangeest JB, Wang C (Eds.). *Understanding Health Literacy: Implications for Medicine and Public Health.* Washington, DC: American Medical Association; 43–53.

National Center for Education Statistics. 2003. *National Assessment of Adult Literacy (NAAL).* Available at http://nces.ed.gov/naal/literacytypes.asp. Accessed September 8, 2010.

Osborne H, 2003. In Other Words . . . Make It Easy . . . Writing Healthcare Forms That Patients Can Understand and Complete. *On Call.* 6(3):16–17. Available at http://www.healthliteracy.com/healthcare-forms. Accessed January 13, 2011.

Osborne H (host). 2010, July 13. Health Literacy from a Literacy Perspective [audio podcast]. *Health Literacy Out Loud,* no. 41. Available at http://www.healthliteracy .com/hlol-literacy-perspective. Accessed January 13, 2011.

Sources to Learn More

Evetts J, Gauthier M. 2005. *Literacy Task Assessment Guide.* National Literacy Secretariat, Human Resources and Skills Development Canada. Ottawa, ON.

Osborne H (host). 2009, December 17. Using Design to Get Readers to Read and Keep Reading [audio podcast]. *Health Literacy Out Loud,* no. 29. Available at http://www .healthliteracy.com/hlol-design-principles. Accessed January 13, 2011.

General Public: Talking with Patients About What They Learn from the Media

STARTING POINTS

Unlike the "old days" when most people learned about health from their doctors, today the general public is nearly bombarded with health and medical stories from television, radio, Internet sites, newspapers, magazines, and other popular media.

While this groundswell of media information can bring beneficial "teaching moments" for patients and their providers, it also creates some challenges. For instance, patients may panic after reading a newspaper article about someone who has the same diagnosis they do. Or they may have unrealistic expectations about a certain treatment and insist they need a particular drug after watching direct-to-consumer (DTC) advertising.

Lisa M. Jones, MD, FACOG, knows a lot about the interplay of medicine and media. She is a practicing gynecologist and interned with the medical division of a major television broadcaster. Jones offers suggestions about how providers can help their patients make sense of information from the media.

STRATEGIES, IDEAS, AND SUGGESTIONS

Here are some suggestions you could put into practice (Osborne 2007):

Pay attention to the news. Jones recommends that providers stay up to date with health reports by periodically checking the news throughout the day.

She explains that media stories are often aired the same day that studies are published. This happens because most medical journals send articles to news outlets ahead of their publication date, "embargoing" them (that is, requesting these stories not be aired) for a defined period of time. In practice, this means that patients may see media stories on medical or health findings before providers have reviewed the research.

Pay attention to the ads. Direct-to-consumer (DTC) advertising about medication is another example of how the popular media can affect clinical practice. Help your patients appreciate the influence of ads, such as how the picture of a cute teddy bear or sleeping baby on the label of children's medication may encourage parents to buy it.

Pay attention to the shows. In addition to news stories and advertising, television shows can impact patients' perceptions of medical care. Many of these create unrealistic expectations about access to care, says Jones. Examples include shows in which the same doctor gives a diagnosis, performs all scans and tests, and also does surgery. Or shows that imply there is always a quick and direct line from symptoms to diagnosis.

Pay attention to spikes in phone calls. In most medical offices, front-desk staff and nurses are the first to speak with patients. Jones asks that everyone working in her office be aware of spikes in the number of calls about certain topics or specific health stories. Here is what she recommends when spikes occur:

- **Prepare a standard office response.** Jones prepares a script for nurses and office staff to give in response to calls about "hot topics." The script might go something like this, "Yes, the study came out yesterday and we know it is in the news. While the journal article is not yet widely available, Dr. Jones is confident that [something from this study that the doctor thinks patients should know now]. Let us make an appointment for you to speak with her in the next week after she has reviewed the article." Jones finds that standard office responses help reassure patients that the situation is not an emergency and offer an acceptable follow-up plan.
- **Research the research.** When Jones hears about a new health story, she not only reads the peer-reviewed research but also investigates the quality of journalism. One of the first sources she consults is the Foundation for Informed Medical Decision Making's Web site, www.healthnewsreview.org. Run by the School of Journalism and Mass Communication at the University of Minnesota, this site uses stringent criteria to grade health stories on a scale of 1 to 5.

- **Refer patients to resources you trust.** Often, patients want to know more about a specific health story. Jones recommends that offices provide lists of credible, accurate resources. Some Web sites that she consistently recommends are: WebMD at www.webmd.com; the Mayo Clinic Web site at http://mayoclinic.com; and ABC News Health at http://abcnews.go.com/Health.

Stories from Practice: Recalling False Information as True

Your grandmother has arthritis and is desperately seeking a cure. She recalls reading that someone (she can't remember who) in some newspaper (she can't recall which one) said that shark cartilage is helpful. You know this is not the case and that using shark cartilage is really just a scam. So you tell her several times, "Grandma, it is not true that shark cartilage helps arthritis." A week later, though, she is even more convinced that shark cartilage is what she needs.

Your grandmother doesn't necessarily have dementia. She simply may be experiencing a memory problem that affects almost everyone. It's common for people to recall false information as true. For people to remember information accurately, they need to recall both the "claim"—the core piece of information—and its "context"—the situation in which they heard it. For most people, remembering the claim is easy, especially if they hear it more than once. Memory of context, however, fades quickly, which means people lose details such as how or where they heard something.

One way to help is by stating information in positive rather than negative ways. When giving instructions with bulleted "do/don't do" lists, phrase information in positive ways whenever possible. This is because readers may remember the gist of a message but not negative words like "don't" or "avoid."

Another way to help is by emphasizing what's true, rather than what's false. Don't start with misinformation even if you intend to correct it. If you must repeat false information, put it in the middle of a document and not at the beginning or end, which are places where people tend to pay most attention.

Source: Osborne (2008).

Television shows can create unrealistic expectations about access to care. Examples include shows in which the same doctor gives a diagnosis, performs all scans and tests, and also does surgery. Or shows that imply there is always a quick and direct line from symptoms to diagnosis. 〝〞

CITATIONS

Osborne H. 2007, January/February. In Other Words . . . Talking About the Media. *On Call*. Available at http://www.healthliteracy.com/media. Accessed January 14, 2011.

Osborne H. 2008, February 28. In Other Words . . . Helping Patients Separate True Health Information from False. *On Call*. Available at http://www.healthliteracy.com/true-false-information. Accessed January 14, 2011.

SOURCES TO LEARN MORE

Frosch DL, Krueger PM, Hornik RC, Cronholm PF, Barg FK. 2007. Creating Demand for Prescription Drugs: A Content Analysis of Television Direct-to-Consumer Advertising. *Annals of Family Medicine*. 5(1):6–13.

Osborne H. 2008, January 10. In Other Words . . . How Memory Affects Health Understanding. *On Call*. Available at http://www.healthliteracy.com/memory. Accessed January 14, 2011.

Osborne H. 2008, December 31. In Other Words . . . Pediatric Cough and Cold Medicine: Helping Patients Make Sense of Information from the FDA. *On Call*. Available at http://www.healthliteracy.com/fda-information. Accessed January 14, 2011.

Skurnik I, Yoon C, Park DC, Schwarz N. 2005. How Warnings About False Claims Become Recommendations. *Journal of Consumer Research*. 31(4):713–724.

Stein K, Zhao L, Crammer C, Gansler T. 2007. Prevalence and Sociodemographic Correlates of Beliefs Regarding Cancer Risks. *Cancer*. 110(5):1139–1148.

Humor and Healing

Health care is admittedly serious business. While there are many conversations about life-and-death issues that cannot and should not be taken lightly, there also are occasions when a dose of humor can help build rapport, facilitate learning, and improve understanding. Indeed, humor is a powerful tool that providers can use to enhance communication and demonstrate compassion and humanity.

STRATEGIES, IDEAS, AND SUGGESTIONS

Here are some ideas you might want to try (Osborne 2003; 2010):

Gauge the other person's sense of humor. Humor includes jokes, riddles, word play, visual gags, and silly objects or cartoons. Consider the other person's learning style, age, culture, and gender when choosing which, if any, type of humor to use. One way to gauge humor is by noting how the person reacts to funny pictures in the room or silly pins you are wearing. Try also to notice the other person's style, such as whether she or he enjoys visual cartoons or prefers word play such as puns and quips. All these ways can serve as signposts about where you can go with this person in terms of humor.

Show humor. If you're not comfortable telling jokes or being silly, you can show humor in quieter ways. For example, in your waiting room you might

Stories from Practice: Humor Connects in Personal and Positive Ways

Karyn Lynn Buxman, RN, MS, is recognized for her expertise in applied and therapeutic humor. She not only was a nurse and is a humorist, but also publishes the *Journal of Nursing Jocularity*.

Buxman and I spoke about humor in health care, and she shared many stories. One that particularly resonated with me was about when she worked as a home health care nurse, caring for a woman with terminal cancer. Buxman visited this family each week. Obviously, the patient and her family appreciated these visits, as they wanted to give Buxman a present.

When asked what she would like, Buxman said she would enjoy hearing a funny story. So the next week, the woman and her husband told Buxman something amusing that their young granddaughter just said. The following week they shared another anecdote. And even as the woman's health declined, every week this family found something lighthearted to share. To me, the lesson of Buxman's story is that humor is a wonderful tool to connect people in personal and positive ways, even during stressful and sad times.

Source: Buxman (2011).

have amusing photos on the wall or display magazines with great cartoons. If your dress code permits, you might show your sense of humor by what you wear—such as colorful neckties, silly pins, or doodads on your stethoscope. In print, too, you can include a dose of humor with clever illustrations or ridiculous examples.

Bridge from humor to teaching. When teaching new concepts or treatment techniques, you might want to use humor in your introduction or as a way of keeping people interested and engaged. For example, you might heighten teenagers' interest in proper nutrition by first showing them a special "food chart for teens." When the teens see refined sugar, fat, caffeine, and salt listed as the four major food groups, they can laugh at how ridiculous this diet is and be more receptive to learning about healthy foods.

If in doubt, don't say it. Humor should be used in small doses and not detract from treatment and care. Certainly there are times when humor is not appropriate, such as when people hear bad news, are angry, or are struggling emotionally. People may need to cry before they can laugh.

Recover when humor backfires. Despite good planning and sensitivity, sometimes humor backfires and is not appropriate or appreciated. If your attempts at being funny fall flat, quickly apologize and let the other person know that you are not trying to be hurtful. In turn, when someone tells you a joke that you find offensive, don't overreact. You might say something like "that's a creative way of looking at things" and then quickly change the subject.

Stories from Practice: Joy and Fun in Our Lives

Izzy Gesell knows a lot about the healing power of humor and play. He sees the value of humor in all his work, whether as a special education teacher, a stand-up comic, or an organizational consultant.

"Humor is not always about being funny. It's about seeing the world from the same perspective as someone else," Gesell explains. He says that people tend to feel more connected and less alone when laughing with others. "Even if you are not naturally funny, there is room to have joy and fun in our lives," says Gesell.

Source: Osborne (2010, April 27).

 Humor is a powerful tool to help people connect in personal and positive ways, even during stressful and sad times. 🙶

CITATIONS

Buxman K. 2011. Telephone interview.

Osborne H. 2003, July/August. In Other Words . . . Adding a Dose of Humor to Your Patient Teaching. *On Call.* Available at http://www.healthliteracy.com/humor. Accessed September 9, 2010.

Osborne H (host). 2010, April 27. The Healing Power of Humor and Play [audio podcast]. *Health Literacy Out Loud,* no. 36. Available at http://healthliteracy.com/hlol-humor-play. Accessed September 8, 2010.

SOURCES TO LEARN MORE

Association for Applied and Therapeutic Humor, http://www.aath.org. Accessed September 8, 2010.

IzzyG & Company, http://www.izzyg.com

Journal of Nursing Jocularity, http://www.journalofnursingjocularity.com.

Karyn Buxman, http://www.karynbuxman.com.

Osborne H (host). 2008, November 17. Jan Potter Talks About Using Humor and Graphics to Convey Health Information [audio podcast]. *Health Literacy Out Loud,* no. 5. Available at http://www.healthliteracy.com/hlol-graphics-humor Accessed September 9, 2010.

What's So Funny About, http://whatssofunnyabout.com

World Laughter Tour, Inc., http://www.worldlaughtertour.com

Interpreters and Translations

STARTING POINTS

Patients need to be knowledgeable about health problems affecting their lives. While learning what to do and why to do it can be a challenging task, this type of communication is even more difficult when patients and providers lack a common language. Language gaps like these are increasingly common. According to a report about U.S. Census Bureau data, more than 55 million people in the United States (about 20 percent of the population) speak a language other than English at home (Shin & Kominski 2010).

Interpreters and translators help bridge language gaps. Interpreters convert the spoken word from one language into another, such as from English to Hindi or from spoken English to American Sign Language (ASL), which is used by many people in the Deaf community. Translators do essentially the same, but with the written word. This can include translating discharge instructions, patient's rights, informed consent documents, medical bills, and even signs or maps that help newcomers find their way around unfamiliar places.

STRATEGIES, IDEAS, AND SUGGESTIONS

Here are some strategies you may find useful when working with interpreters or preparing translated materials (Gillispie 2011; Osborne 2000, July; 2003, June; 2003, November/December; 2006, January/February):

Interpreters

Professional medical interpreters are the best source of help, as they not only are trained in medical vocabulary but are also instructed in how to maintain neutrality, adhere to confidentiality, and not impose personal views. When onsite-trained medical interpreters are not available, organizations might engage over-the-phone interpretation services like Language Line (www.languageline.com).

There may be times when providers seek language help from bilingual volunteers, perhaps staff members or people in the patient's family. But this can lead to problems, as when an untrained interpreter inadvertently misinterprets a term or interjects his or her opinion. Another concern is about violations of privacy and confidentiality. And children especially should not interpret for their parents or other family members—as doing so can place them in the midst of health conversations they shouldn't be a part of.

Stories from Practice: Interpreters Help Clarify Problems

"Lydia," an elderly Russian-speaking woman, was in the hospital recovering from surgery. Late one evening, Lydia was making motions on her chest. The night nurse wasn't sure if Lydia was having chest pain or was trying to tell her something, so she paged the medical interpreter to clarify.

The interpreter asked the patient if she was having chest pain. Lydia responded, "My heart hurts because my daughter hasn't come to visit me, and I'm feeling sad." Once she had that piece of information, the nurse was able to appropriately intervene and help Lydia deal with her sadness.

Source: Osborne (2000).

Help patients feel welcome. When you do not share a common language or way of communicating, you can create a feeling of welcome by greeting patients in their native tongue or using ASL to sign "hello." Even if you mangle pronunciation, it is still evident that at least you cared enough to try.

Allow sufficient time. Conversations may take two to three times longer when using interpreters. Ideally, allow sufficient time in your schedule to meet briefly with an interpreter before and after speaking with the patient.

Look at and speak directly to the patient, not the interpreter. You not only show respect this way but also can notice a patient's nonverbal cues. When working with an ASL interpreter, the interpreter should sit a little behind and to the side of the health provider. This way, the patient can see both the provider and interpreter in the same visual field. The provider, in turn, can listen to the interpreter while looking directly at the patient.

Provide translated tools of basic phrases. There invariably will be times when you need to communicate with non-English-speaking patients and a qualified interpreter is not available. In these instances, tools (booklets, cards, and software or other electronic applications) with translations of basic phrases might help. They can include basic questions like "Are you hungry?" or "Are you in pain?" with the choice of several responses including "Yes," "No," and "I don't know." To use these tools, however, patients must be able to read in their native languages and the phrases must be accurately translated.

Communicate your message in alternative ways. Here are some examples:

- Make simple drawings, such as to indicate when to call the doctor or how to measure a medicine.
- Use an anatomic model to demonstrate how to do a self-care activity.
- Use visuals to rate pain. An example is the *Wong-Baker FACES Pain Rating Scale*. On this 10-point scale, patients can express the intensity of their pain by pointing to a facial expression ranging from smiling (no hurt) to crying (hurts worst). Learn more at http://www .wongbakerfaces.org/.
- Provide health information in audio, Web-video, and other formats. One of my favorite resources for health information in many languages and multiple formats is Healthy Roads Media (www .healthyroadsmedia.org).

Appreciate differences in body language. Beyond words, some gestures and body language are not universally understood. While feelings of anger and happiness may look alike around the world, even "yes" and "no" are sometimes communicated in different ways. In the United States for example, it is assumed that a nod means "yes," while in other languages, a nod may simply mean "I hear what you said." A good source to learn about integrating cultural information into clinical practice is Ethnomed (http:// ethnomed.org/).

Notice signs of difficulty. Regardless of language differences, it is the health provider's responsibility to make sure that medical information is communicated accurately. If you sense that there is a problem, such as lengthy conversations between the interpreter and patient and only one-word answers to you, withdraw from the situation and speak privately with the interpreter to make sure the message is being communicated correctly.

Verify understanding. Just as when communicating in English, ask patients to tell you, via interpreters, how they understand information and instructions. Ask questions that require more than simple "yes" or "no" answers. Instead, ask open-ended questions like "How would you take this medicine?" rather than "Do you understand what to do?"

Translations

Develop and test materials with intended readers. Just like all other forms of communication, translated materials must be presented in ways readers can understand and relate to. One of the best ways to accomplish this is by working collaboratively with those who represent the intended audience. This includes working together to develop ideas, deciding about word choice and illustrations, and then testing drafts along the way.

For practices with very diverse populations, Mary Alice Gillispie, MD, of Healthy Roads Media suggests partnering across organizations and with academic centers to help share the load and high cost of developing translated materials. To reduce duplication of effort, Gillispie recommends tailoring or customizing already translated materials from trusted sources such as MedlinePlus (www.nlm.nih.gov/medlineplus).

If you want to change materials that are not in the public domain, make sure to get permission to do so from the content author. In Gillispie's experience, "Just about everyone working in this area is very willing to have their materials customized to be more useful for local settings and appreciates hearing that their resources are helpful."

Simplify your message before translation. Rather than insist on a literal (word-for-word) translation, work with a professional translator or community team to make needed adaptations for linguistic and cultural differences. Confirm that the translated document is accurate by asking others to "proof" that this version is correct. Make sure that the typist is also familiar with the language being used. Even well-translated documents can lose their meaning when important accent marks are omitted or misplaced. Keep in mind that professional translators are not necessarily health experts; that job belongs to you.

Inform patients about translations. I've seen many healthcare documents with statements like, "Please let us know if you need this booklet in [x language]." Ironically, sometimes these statements are only in English. Instead, make sure to translate such statements into the language of your readers.

Decide whether to put two languages in one document. Sometimes there are requests to put two or more languages in the same document. This may mean to have one language at the top of a page and the other language on the bottom, or to have one language upside-down from the other. While these layouts may work well for readers, they can present design challenges. For example, English is a tighter language than most. This means it takes up less space than a language like Spanish, which is about 20 to 30 percent larger than English. As a result, text may look crowded with two languages on the same page.

Use meaningful examples and illustrations. Translated documents usually include more than just words. Make sure that the examples and illustrations you use are consistent with the culture, age, and interests of your readers. For example, when translating a nutrition brochure you might chose whether to mention tacos, egg rolls, crepes, or blintzes.

Interpreters convert the spoken word from one language into another, such as from English to Hindi or from spoken English to American Sign Language (ASL), which is used by many people in the Deaf community. Translators do essentially the same, but with the written word. **"**

CITATIONS

Osborne H. 2000, July. In Other Words . . . When You Truly Need to Find Other Words . . . Working with Medical Interpreters. *On Call.* Available at http://www .healthliteracy.com/medical-interpreters. Accessed September 12, 2010.

Osborne H. 2003, June. In Other Words. . . Communicating About Health with ASL. *On Call.* 6(6):16–17. Available at http://www.healthliteracy.com/american-sign-language. Accessed September 12, 2010.

Osborne H. 2003, November/December. In Other Words. . . Communicating About Health with New Immigrants. *On Call.* 6(10):16–17. Available at http://www .healthliteracy.com/new-immigrants. Accessed September 12, 2010.

Osborne H. 2006, January/February. In Other Words . . . Actions Can Speak as Clearly as Words. *On Call.* Available at http://healthliteracy.com/actions Accessed June 16, 2011.

Shin HB, Kominski RA. 2010, April. *Language Use in the United States: 2007.* U.S. Census Bureau. Available at http://www.census.gov/prod/2010pubs/acs-12 .pdf. Accessed September 12, 2010.

Sources to Learn More

American Translators Association, www.atanet.org

The Cross Cultural Health Care Program, www.xculture.org

Dollinger RK. 1992. *Pocket Medical Spanish*. Van Nuys, CA: Booksmythe.

Flores G, Laws MB, Mayo SJ, Zuckerman B, Abreu M, Medina L, et al. 2003. Errors in Medical Interpretation and Their Potential Clinical Consequences in Pediatric Encounters. *Pediatrics.* 111(1):6–14.

Gillispie MA, 2011. Personal communication.

Kelly N. 2008. The Voice on the Other End of the Phone. *Health Affairs* 27(6): 1701–1706.

Morales LS, Elliiott M, Weech-Maldonado R, Hays RD. 2006. The Impact of Interpreters on Parents' Experiences with Ambulatory Care for Their Children. *Medical Care Research and Review.* 63(1):110–128.

National Council on Interpreting in Health Care. 2007. *FAQs for Healthcare Professionals.* Available at http://www.ncihc.org/mc/page.do?sitePageId=101286&orgId=ncihc. Accessed September 12, 2010.

Osborne H (host). 2010, January 26. A Participatory Approach for Communicating with Diverse Audiences [audio podcast]. *Health Literacy Out Loud,* no. 31. Available at http://www.healthliteracy.com/hlol-participatory-approach. Accessed January 18, 2011.

Solomon FM, Eberl-Lefko AC, Michaels M, Macario E, Tesauro G, Rowland JH. 2005. Development of a Linguistically and Culturally Appropriate Booklet for Latino Cancer Survivors: Lessons Learned. *Health Promotion Practice.* 6(4):405–413.

U.S. Department of Health & Human Services, Office of Minority Health, http://minorityhealth.hhs.gov

Jargon, Acronyms, and Other Troublesome Words

STARTING POINTS

Health professionals spend many years learning a new, specialized language. It is usually quite effective to use as a sort of shorthand with colleagues and coworkers. But to patients and other outsiders, such specialized language may be unclear. Here are examples of some troublesome types of words:

Jargon. Medical jargon refers to technical terms and phrases or words used in special, idiosyncratic ways. While these terms are familiar and helpful to health professionals, patients and families may not understand jargon in the same way. For example, in health care the term "unremarkable" generally means "you're fine," while the term "positive" (as in "your blood test came back positive for [x]") may mean you're not. For sure, that is not how most laypeople understand these words.

Abbreviations, acronyms, and initialisms. These refer to shortened ways of referring to longer, more complicated terms. They can be very efficient when talking with peers or entering data into medical charts. Abbreviations are usually shortened versions of longer words, such as "prep" for "preparation." Acronyms and initialisms usually take the first letters from each word in a phrase to create something new. Sometimes they sound familiar like "CAT" for "computed/computerized axial tomography." Other times, they create a new "word" (which really isn't a word) like "ADL," which stands for "activities of daily living."

Homonyms. These are words that sound alike and may or may not be spelled the same way, but have very different meanings. Health care uses a lot of homonyms like "stool," "gait," and "dressing." Be aware that patients can easily misinterpret homonyms. As with all new words, make sure to clarify exactly what you mean.

Idioms. These are phrases that mean something quite different from their actual words. Generally, idioms have special meaning to people from a certain region or culture. This meaning, however, may be unfamiliar to outsiders. Because most health materials are written for a general (not local) reading audience, try to avoid using idioms like "feeling blue" and "heads up."

"Simple" words that aren't so simple. Sometimes even commonly used words like "may," "might," and "suggest" are difficult to understand. This often happens when describing risk. While the phrase "this treatment might help" can mean to a scientist that there is no conclusive evidence, it can be interpreted as "this treatment will help" to a patient desperate for hope.

Stories from Practice: Abbreviations in the ED or ER

Imagine what it is like to be suddenly injured or ill. You or your family member calls 911. **EMT**s arrive and take you to the nearest **ER** or **ED**. You or your family member is given a lot of paperwork, including **HIPAA** notification. The doctors and nurses say you need an **IV**, **MRI**, and **CT** scan. And all this before you are admitted to the **ICU**.

Now replay this scenario and imagine being someone who never needed emergency care before. Maybe you also are new to this country and speak only a limited amount of English. You now not only are dealing with pain and uncertainty but also must fully comprehend a new language of healthcare abbreviations (shortened words and phrases) and acronyms (new terms, usually made from the first letters in a series of words).

Source: Osborne (2008).

STRATEGIES, IDEAS, AND SUGGESTIONS

Here are some suggestions about choosing the right words (Osborne 2008):

Make sure the meanings of acronyms are clear.

- Choose only those acronyms and abbreviations that benefit the other person, not just you. For instance, there may be no need to introduce an acronym if you use the term only once. For instance, does your audience really need to know that the acronym for "National Institutes of Health" is "NIH"? Maybe yes, maybe no. My recommendation is that you make choices about acronyms based on what matters to the audience.
- If an acronym is really needed, help by explaining its meaning. Put either the acronym or full term in parentheses alongside the other, such as "BP (blood pressure)." While some editors may disagree, for the sake of clarity and understanding I recommend deciding in each instance whether to put the full form of the word or its acronym first. I tend to write the most commonly used term first, and then either the acronym or full wording.
- Readers might sometimes benefit from a clear explanation rather than the acronym spelled out. For instance, "IV, a needle that goes into your arm."
- Acronyms can have different meanings depending on where and how they are used. For example, "AAA" can stand for the American Automobile Association, the Area Agency on Aging, or an aortic abdominal aneurysm. Provide context to help readers determine which acronym you mean.

Be aware of pronunciation. Acronyms and initialisms are pronounced differently. For example, "HIPAA" (Health Insurance Portability and Accountability Act) is an acronym and pronounced as a single word. But "CHF" (congestive heart failure) is an initialism and pronounced as three distinct letters.

Write out full directions rather than abbreviations. This is particularly important for dosing instructions. While clinicians know the meaning of terms such as QD or SID (once a day), QOD or EOD (every other day), BID (twice a day), and TID (three times a day), patients may not. Clearly explain what to do, giving instructions like "Take this pill two times a day—one pill at breakfast and one pill at dinner time." It can help even more to specify the time, such as "8:00 in the morning and 6:00 at night."

Stories from Practice: Understanding the Meaning of Terms

Jeanne McGee, PhD, author of *Toolkit for Making Written Material Clear and Effective*, does a lot of consumer testing of written material. She recalls interviewing several patients about a handout on hemoglobin A1c (or simply, A1c), which is a type of blood glucose testing.

McGee asked patients about the meaning of certain words and terms. To her surprise, one person said that he thought that "A1c" stood for "airman first class." Another pronounced it "alc" (as in alcoholic) in part because the font made it look more like the letter "l" rather than the numeral "1." McGee subsequently changed the font and rewrote the term as "A-1-C."

McGee also added a pronunciation guide ("A-one-see"). "Some acronyms are pronounced in weird ways and others are pronounced just by saying each letter in turn. It's friendly to provide guidance when pronunciation is not straightforward," says McGee.

Source: McGee (2011)

Avoid gobbledygook. Messages are clearer when you avoid jargon or define terms in ways your intended audience can understand. One clue that you might be using problematic words is by noticing any squiggly lines that appear while you type (if you haven't turned off the spelling and grammar check in your word processor). On my computer, this happens when words are either misspelled or so rare that basic dictionaries do not recognize them. Squiggly lines like these might indicate that your words will be hard for another person to understand.

> *Medical jargon refers to technical terms and phrases or words used in special, idiosyncratic ways. While these terms are familiar and helpful to health professionals, patients and families may not understand jargon in the same way.*

CITATIONS

McGee J. 2011. Personal communication.

Osborne H. 2008, April 10. In Other Words . . . Abbreviations, Acronyms, and Other Healthcare Shorthand. *On Call*. Available at http://www.healthliteracy.com/abbreviations-acronyms. Accessed January 16, 2011.

SOURCES TO LEARN MORE

Medical Library Association. 2007. *Deciphering Medspeak: Medspeak in Plain Language.* Available at http://www.mlanet.org/resources/medspeak/medspeak_plain .html. Accessed January 17, 2011.

Osborne H. 2000, November. In Other Words . . . When It's Time to Choose . . . Thinking About the Right Words. *On Call.* Available at http://www.healthliteracy .com/choosing-the-right-words. Accessed January 17, 2011.

Osborne H. 2004, March. In Other Words . . . The Ethics of Simplicity *On Call.* Available at http://www.healthliteracy.com/ethics-of-simplicity. Accessed August 1, 2010.

The Plain Language Action and Information Network (PLAIN), www.plainlanguage .gov

U.S. Department of Health and Human Services, Centers for Medicare and Medicaid Services, by Jeanne McGee of McGee & Evers Consulting. 2010. *Toolkit for Making Written Material Clear and Effective.* Available at http://www.cms.gov/ WrittenMaterialsToolkit/. Accessed January 8, 2011.

Know Your Audience: Children and Youth

STARTING POINTS

Health literacy is a factor for children, their parents or other caregivers, and pediatric health care providers. Each has an important part to play in helping children be healthy. As succinctly stated in "Health Literacy and Children: Introduction" in the journal *Pediatrics*, "What is most complex and distinct about pediatric health literacy is that it must be considered in terms of parents' or caregivers' health literacy as well as the children's own health literacy (which is evolving as children grow, learn, and develop)" (Abrams, Klass, & Dreyer 2009).

STRATEGIES, IDEAS, AND SUGGESTIONS

Jessica Hennessey, RN, CPNP, is a pediatric nurse practitioner. Hennessey shares strategies for engaging children and their parents in health conversations (Osborne 2001):

Talk to the child about health. Hennessey says that when a child is an active participant in the exam, he or she is likely to be cooperative and to give honest information. So she usually speaks directly to the child, inviting the parents to "chime in" as necessary. In a well checkup, for example, Hennessey might ask Johnny if he wears a seat belt "all of the time" or "some of the time." While the parent might insist that he always wears a seat belt, Johnny might admit that he sometimes forgets to buckle up when

Stories from Practice: Health Literacy Acquisition

Mary Ann Abrams, MD, MPH, FAAP, is a health literacy champion, pediatrician, and co-editor of *Plain Language Pediatrics: Health Literacy Strategies and Communication Resources for Common Pediatric Topics.* She talked with me about age-appropriate acquisition of health literacy skills. Abrams explains that this begins when toddlers learn to name body parts and preschoolers start doing self-care tasks with supervision, such as applying sunscreen and brushing their teeth. With guidance, school-age children can begin to assume greater responsibility, such as reading nutrition labels or using an asthma inhaler. Teenagers then can participate even more independently as they transition from being pediatric to adult patients.

Abrams recommends, "Find age-appropriate ways for children to participate in health. An example is asking a 6-year-old to put a mark on a chart for each time she eats fruits and vegetables. Doing so not only helps the child acquire health literacy skills but also models a way for parents and caregivers to engage the child in healthy actions."

Abrams suggests using principles of motivational interviewing to gauge how confident the child, parent, or caregiver is in following through with an agreed-upon action. For instance, after discussing healthy snack options she might ask a young teenager, "On a scale of 1 to 10, how sure are you that you will eat yogurt instead of chips every time you have a snack?" If the response is low, Abrams and the child may come up with a more realistic option that can result in success and build self-efficacy. Abrams says to use the teach-back technique to confirm that key messages are correctly understood. For instance, after discussing nutrition with a teenager, she may ask, "What will you say to your friends about what you are ordering the next time you go out to eat?"

Source: Abrams (2011).

going to the store. Hennessey takes advantage of such a response to talk about the importance of consistent seat-belt use.

Prepare the child for medical procedures. Communication can be difficult when a child is sick. Not only does the child feel ill, but he or she might also need to have an unpleasant medical procedure performed. When this is the case, Hennessey uses humor and real-life examples to help prepare the child for the procedure. When Mary needs a throat culture, for example, Hennessey might first show her what a swab looks like and let her feel the soft tip. Sometimes she might even let Mary try to take a culture on a doll.

Encourage laughter. Laughing often breaks down communication barriers and can go a long way toward relaxing children and their parents. Engage children in conversation by talking about their favorite TV character or pop singer. Try to play games or use puppets as part of an exam. When listening to a child's breathing, for example, you can ask a child to blow on a pinwheel or pretend to blow out candles on a birthday cake. By encouraging laughter, Hennessey says, "I get what I need and the child is having fun."

Teach in ways that children and their parents or caregivers can learn. This includes putting unfamiliar concepts into context, as for a new diagnosis

---

Stories from Practice: Reach Out and Read

Reach Out and Read is one of my favorite organizations. I had the privilege of interviewing Perri Klass, MD, FAAP, National Medical Director of Reach Out and Read, for a *Health Literacy Out Loud* podcast. As described on its Web site, Reach Out and Read is a "nonprofit initiative that promotes early literacy and school readiness in pediatric exam rooms nationwide."

The Web site outlines three ways Reach Out and Read accomplishes this goal:

- "In the exam room, doctors and nurses speak with parents about the importance of reading aloud to their young children every day, and offer age-appropriate tips and encouragement.
- The pediatric primary care provider gives every child 6 months through 5 years old a new, developmentally appropriate book to take home and keep.
- In the waiting room, displays, information, and books create a literacy-rich environment. Where possible, volunteers read to the children, modeling for parents the pleasures—and techniques—of reading aloud."

Source: Reach Out and Read, www.reachoutandread.org; Osborne (2011).

or medication. It also means using familiar wording like a "stuffy, runny nose" rather than "nasal congestion."

An excellent resource about effective communication is the book *Plain Language Pediatrics: Health Literacy Strategies and Communication Resources for Common Pediatric Topics*. It includes 25 patient education materials for various ages covering acute, chronic, and preventive topics. These handouts are written in plain language and available in English and Spanish (Abrams & Dreyer 2009).

 Find age-appropriate ways for children to participate in health. An example is asking a 6-year-old to put a mark on a chart for each time she eats fruits and vegetables. Doing so not only helps the child acquire health literacy skills but also models a way for parents and caregivers to engage the child in healthy actions.

CITATIONS

Abrams MA. 2011. Interview with author.

Abrams MA, Dreyer BP. 2009. *Plain Language Pediatrics: Health Literacy Strategies and Communication Resources for Common Pediatric Topics*. Elk Grove, IL: American Academy of Pediatrics.

Abrams MA, Klass P, Dreyer BP. 2009, September. Health Literacy and Children: Introduction. *Pediatrics* 124(Suppl.):S262–S264.

Osborne H. 2001, March. In Other Words . . . Start Where They Are . . . Communicating with Children and Their Families About Health and Illness. *On Call*. Available at http://www.healthliteracy.com/children-and-families Accessed January 21, 2011.

Osborne H (host). 2011, January 25. Reach Out and Read: Encouraging Literacy and Health Literacy from Childhood On [audio podcast]. *Health Literacy Out Loud*, no. 52. Available at http://healthliteracy.com/hlol-reach-out-and-read Accessed July 23, 2011.

SOURCES TO LEARN MORE

Davis TC, Mayeaux EJ, Fredrickson D, Bocchini JA Jr, Jackson RH, Murphy PW. 1994. Reading Ability of Parents Compared with Reading Level of Pediatric Patient Education Materials. *Pediatrics*. 93(3):460.

Sanders LM, Federuci S, Klass P, Abrams MA, Dreyer B. 2009. Literacy and Child Health: A Systematic Review. *Archives of Pediatrics and Adolescent Medicine* 163(2):131–140.

Tran TP, Robinson LM, Keebler JR, Walker RA, Wadman MC. 2008. Health Literacy Among Parents of Pediatric Patients. *Western Journal of Emergency Medicine*. 9(3):130–134.

Know Your Audience: Culture and Language

STARTING POINTS

Accessing, using, and understanding the U.S. healthcare system is difficult for almost everyone. But for people who speak limited English or come from other cultures, these tasks might seem impossible. For example, people may not know how to access appropriate healthcare services. Or they might not understand new and complicated medical terminology. It may well be that they find all these tasks difficult and confusing. As the U.S. population grows increasingly diverse, situations like these are becoming more common.

In terms of language, it can take people many years to become fluent. With limited English, people may have sufficient social language to talk about the food or weather. But until they are truly fluent, they might have difficulty discussing "how" and "why" concepts common in health conversations.

Culture, too, impacts how people understand and make sense of health information. Whether born and brought up in the United States or somewhere else in the world, people bring their own experiences, values, customs, and logic to each situation. For example, those from regions where health resources are scarce may not understand why screening tests such as mammograms, Pap smears, and blood pressure checks are routinely recommended.

Despite cultural and linguistic differences, health providers must communicate in ways that all of their patients can understand. This is more than just good patient care. It is also the law. Under Title IV of the U.S. Civil Rights Act of 1964, health professionals are responsible for bridging communication gaps with patients who speak other languages and come from other countries.

Stories from Practice: Health Care from a Native American Perspective

In a *Health Literacy Out Loud* podcast, Linda Burhansstipanov, MSPH, DrPH (known to many as "Linda B"), of the Cherokee Nation of Oklahoma talked about health care from a Native American perspective. We began by discussing terminology. Burhansstipanov said that, as with other sensitive issues, acceptable wording depends who you are talking to. She said that some tribes prefer the term Native American, while others prefer the terms American Indian, First Nation, or indigenous people.

Burhansstipanov's research and teaching focus on cancer screening, early detection, and treatment. Beyond the usual teaching challenges, she said that communication is often even harder because, until recently, cancer was not openly addressed in the Native community. She explained that some people felt that using the word "cancer" spreads the "cancer spirit." For a while, instead of using the word "cancer," people referred to it as "the disease for which there is no cure."

Burhansstipanov also talked about framing cancer messages within a cultural context. She used the example of mammograms. Rather than talking about personal health benefits of mammograms, she recommends framing these in terms of the family. Burhansstipanov offered examples such as, "Have a mammogram to show your family how a well woman behaves," or "Have a mammogram to be alive to tell your stories to the next generation."

Source: Osborne (2010, August 24).

STRATEGIES, IDEAS, AND SUGGESTIONS

Here are some helpful strategies (Osborne 1999; 2000; 2003; 2009, July 13; 2010, August 24):

Create a welcoming atmosphere. Welcome patients by displaying multicultural artifacts, globes, and worldwide maps. Translated signs are important as well. Greet patients in their native languages and ask how to pronounce their names correctly. Even if your pronunciation is less than perfect, you have conveyed a willingness to communicate despite linguistic differences.

Work with interpreters and translators.

- *Interpreters* work with the spoken word, communicating what one person says in words that another person understands. When talking about important health information, work with trained medical interpreters rather than bilingual family, friends, or volunteers. Trained interpreters are educated in medical vocabulary, ethics, and confidentiality and can also serve as "cultural brokers" to present information in keeping with the other person's beliefs and practices.
- *Translators* work with the written word, taking information from one language to another. Beyond words, translated materials should be culturally appropriate and include graphics and examples that readers can accept and relate to. (Read more in "Interpreters and Translations," starting on page 81.)

Ask who makes decisions. In some cultures, patients are not the ones to make health decisions. Find out whether the patient, someone in his or her family, or a designated decision-maker accepts this responsibility. Include this person when discussing diagnostic information and treatment options.

Speak at a slower pace. When talking with people who speak limited English, focus on essential, need-to-know skills and behaviors rather than nice-to-know background information. Speak at a slower pace, pausing for two or three seconds after asking questions or giving new information. But do not speak louder just because people have limited English—this can come across as sounding angry and does nothing to improve communication.

When possible, use common words. Examples include using the word "cancer" rather than "oncology," or "kidney doctor" and not "nephrologist." Avoid medical jargon and acronyms like "BP" when you can just as simply say "blood pressure."

Be aware that some concepts, treatments, and tests may not be able to be translated into a single word. This includes terms for some treatments and tests, such as "genetic testing" and "psychiatric counseling." It may take many translated words to explain their meaning clearly.

Stories from Practice: Be Aware of Unfamiliar Concepts

According to Mary Alice Gillispie, MD, of Healthy Roads Media, some health concepts are not universally understood. This includes concepts like preventive care. Gillispie says, "Going to the doctor and being treated for something when you have no symptoms (for example, high blood pressure) is not the norm in less developed parts of the world."

Gillispie adds, "This means that extra effort will sometimes need to be made to help patients understand why a treatment is needed. Without this understanding, the chance that patients will seek out and follow treatment plans is low."

Source: Gillispie (2011).

Pay attention to nonverbal language. Whether you communicate through an interpreter or talk directly with patients, pay as much attention to nonverbal communication as you do to words. Notice the volume and speed at which people speak, and pay attention to their silences, as well. Look also at posture, gestures, and eye contact. Be cautious, however, about making assumptions. In some cultures it is considered rude to look another person in the eye. Likewise, a nod does not always indicate agreement. Sometimes a nod simply means, "I hear what you are saying."

Invite questions. Many patients find it hard to ask questions. It can be even more difficult when people have been taught it is disrespectful to question those in authority. You can help by inviting, encouraging, and even modeling good questions. Burhansstipanov recommends making a statement like, "It's okay for you to ask me a question." She adds that some Indian Health Service clinics also put up posters with suggested questions to ask. (Read more in "Question Asking," starting on page 167.)

Find additional ways to communicate your health message. This can include pictographs (simple line drawings that show ideas or actions), demonstrations, stories, and metaphors. Consider "hands-on" practice as well. For example, instead of just telling patients how to take a new liquid medication, use an actual dosing spoon to demonstrate what to do and then have patients re-demonstrate how they would do it.

Confirm understanding. When communicating with patients who speak other languages and come from other countries, do not assume that a nod and a smile necessarily mean that your message is understood. To confirm understanding, ask an open-ended question such as, "How will you . . . ?" rather than a yes/no question like, "Do you know how to . . . ?" When it appears that the other person does not understand, find other ways to communicate the same message. (Read more in "Confirming Understanding: Teach-Back," starting on page 41.)

Stories from Practice: The Hesperian Foundation Creates Books Congruent with Specific Cultures

The Hesperian Foundation, based in Berkeley, California, designs and promotes materials oriented toward people in developing countries who have limited access to education and health care. They produce many acclaimed books, including *Where There Is No Doctor*.

In a *Health Literacy Out Loud* podcast, I spoke with Curt Wands-Bourdoiseau, who is a physician assistant serving as the project manager for a major rewrite of this book. He spoke about strategies to create books congruent with specific cultures:

- Begin with the reader's experience of illness, rather than pathophysiology.
- Explain information in a very respectful tone. Encourage people to make use of their great knowledge about life around them.
- Include familiar pictures and simple drawings. To show the passage of time, you might have drawings of sun-up (morning), full sun (noon), and moon (night).
- Provide cultural or ethnic context. This could be showing people squatting on the ground around a campfire rather than sitting on chairs around a table.
- Maintain simple language. For instance, write "short of breath," not "dyspnea."
- Develop the book with community members. Ask community members about important information to include, and get their feedback throughout the writing process. Their input is in addition to, not instead of, input from health professionals.

Sources: Hesperian Foundation, www.hesperian.org; Osborne (2009, July 13).

Whether born and brought up in the United States or somewhere else in the world, people bring their own experiences, values, customs, and logic to each situation. For example, those from regions where health resources are scarce may not understand why screening tests such as mammograms, Pap smears, and blood pressure checks are routinely recommended. ""

CITATIONS

Gillespie MA. 2011. Personal communication.

Osborne H. 1999. In Other Words . . . Communicating with People from Other Cultures. *On Call.* 2(8):42–43. Available at http://www.healthliteracy.com/other-cultures. Accessed January 23, 2011.

Osborne H. 2000. In Other Words . . . It Takes More Than Just Words . . . Culturally and Linguistically Appropriate Materials. *On Call.* 3(4):34–35. http://www.healthliteracy.com/culturally-linguistically-appropriate-materials. Accessed January 23, 2011.

Osborne H. 2000. In Other Words . . . When You Truly Need to Find Other Words . . . Working with Medical Interpreters. *On Call.* 3(7):38–39. http://www.healthliteracy.com/medical-interpreters. Accessed October 15, 2010.

Osborne H. 2003. In Other Words . . . Communicating About Health with New Immigrants. *On Call.* 6(10):16–17. Available at http://www.healthliteracy.com/new-immigrants. Accessed October 15, 2010.

Osborne H (host). 2009, July 13. Developing Healthcare Materials with and for Village Health Workers [audio podcast]. *Health Literacy Out Loud,* no. 18. Available at http://healthliteracy.com/hlol-hesperian. Accessed January 23, 2011.

Osborne H (host). 2010, August 24. Health Communication from a Native American Perspective [audio podcast]. *Health Literacy Out Loud,* no. 44. Available at http://healthliteracy.com/hlol-native-american. Accessed October 12, 2010.

SOURCES TO LEARN MORE

Committee on Communication for Behavior Change in the 21st Century: Improving the Health of Diverse Populations, Board on Neuroscience and Behavioral Health. Institute of Medicine of the National Academies. 2002. *Speaking of Health: Assessing Health Communication Strategies for Diverse Populations.* Washington, DC: National Academies Press.

Fadiman A. 1997. *The Spirit Catches You and You Fall Down: A Hmong Child, Her American Doctors, and the Collision of Two Cultures.* New York: Noonday Press.

Healthy Roads Media, www.healthyroadsmedia.org

Johnstone MJ, Kanitsaki O. 2006. Culture, Language, and Patient Safety: Making the Link. *International Journal for Quality in Health Care* 18(5):383–388.

Kleinman A. 1989. *The Illness Narratives: Suffering, Healing, and the Human Condition.* New York: Basic Books.

Lipson JG, Dibble SL, Minarik PA (eds.). 1996. *Culture and Nursing Care: A Pocket Guide.* San Francisco: UCSF Nursing Press.

McKinney J, Kurtz-Rossi S. 2000. *Culture, Health, and Literacy: A Guide to Health Education Materials for Adults with Limited English Literacy Skills.* Boston: World Education. Available at http://healthliteracy.worlded.org/docs/culture/index .html. Accessed October 15, 2010.

National Archives. n.d. *Teaching with Documents: The Civil Rights Act of 1964 and the Equal Employment Opportunity Commission.* Available at http://www.archives.gov/ education/lessons/civil-rights-act/. Accessed January 23, 2011.

Native American Cancer Research, www.natamcancer.org

U.S. Census Bureau. n.d. *United States Census 2010.* Available at http://2010.census .gov/2010census. Accessed January 23, 2011.

Know Your Audience: Emotions and Cognition

STARTING POINTS

As all of us who have ever been patients or caregivers know, health care is filled with emotion. When we, or those we love and care for, are ill or injured, our emotions can override even the best of communications.

At these times, even seemingly routine medical events can raise our level of anxiety. And when there is a new diagnosis, an urgent need to make a treatment decision, perhaps along with memory loss or cognitive challenges, communication that was already difficult is now even harder.

STRATEGIES, IDEAS, AND SUGGESTIONS

Here are some suggestions you might put into practice (Osborne 2005, May/June; 2005, October; 2008):

When People Are Anxious or Angry

- **Find a private place to talk.** Whenever possible, take the upset patient or family member aside and speak privately about his or her concerns. If it is not possible to go to a separate space, create more privacy by closing curtains, shutting doors, or repositioning chairs.

> ### Stories from Practice: Turning Down the Heat of Anxiety
>
> A 73-year-old man was scheduled for surgery to confirm a cancer diagnosis. He and his wife arrived on time for early morning surgery. But soon after, they were told that the surgery was delayed until early afternoon. By mid-afternoon, they were told that—due to many unexpected surgical emergencies—the surgery would be postponed for one day.
>
> Already anxious about his diagnosis and upcoming surgery, the patient and his wife were irate that surgery was cancelled. The unit staff, nurse manager, and physician all tried to calm the family, keeping them abreast of pertinent information and offering support and reassurance. They also admitted the patient to the hospital so that he would not have to go home that night.
>
> However, the next morning, the wife was even angrier. She seemed to complain about everything, including the temperature of her husband's hospital room. The unit staff asked the patient advocate to intervene. When the patient advocate met with the wife, she began by asking, "What can I do to help you get through this day?" The wife talked about her frustration with the excessive heat in her husband's room.
>
> The patient advocate calmly and efficiently addressed this concern. When she realized the solution required more than just turning down the thermostat, she asked a maintenance worker to meet with the patient's wife. The wife calmed down as soon as she heard an explanation of what was wrong, thanking the patient advocate for her assistance. It was only then that she started to share her real fears about her husband's upcoming surgery.
>
> *Source:* Osborne (2005, October).

- **Choose your words carefully.** Avoid using judgment phrases. It can minimize a patient's experience when health professionals say that a procedure has been delayed for "only" a day, or that he or she is "just" having gall bladder surgery. Appreciate also that when people are anxious, they may only comprehend part of what you are saying. Be prepared to repeat information, offering a pad and pencil so that the patient or family member can take notes and jot down questions.

- **Consider your nonverbal language.** Smile and approach patients and families in a calm manner. Help patients relax by speaking audibly, but softly. Attitude can also make a huge difference. As said by one nurse who earns high praise from patients and families, "It isn't anything magical I do. I'm just nice to patients."
- **Listen, and let the patient talk.** Don't argue, even if you know you are right. Listen to what patients or family members have to say—they might calm down simply by being able to share their concerns. Do not insist on meaningful conversation when patients and families are not ready.
- **Be aware of your own feelings and limitations.** Health professionals are not immune to anxiety or anger. When you find yourself in an upsetting situation or are having a bad day, talk with your colleagues or supervisor. Let others help you brainstorm ways to improve communication.

When Communicating Sad or Bad News

- **Develop rapport.** Find a way to quickly establish rapport and a trusting bond with patients, families, or clients you've just met. Steven Grossman, MD, PhD, is an oncologist. One way he develops rapport is by finding out how much information people already have. To do this, he uses open-ended questions such as, "What is your understanding of what you have?" While one person might say, "I think I have cancer and you'll tell me the rest," another may talk about the Internet printouts she brought to the appointment.
- **Communicate the information people need in ways they understand.** The standard of care for Grossman is to openly discuss diagnosis, prognosis, and treatment options with his patients. Within this standard, however, he uses clinical judgment to decide how to present this information. While one patient may want to know mostly about prognosis, another may be much more eager to discuss treatment options. Regardless of the news, Grossman always finds something positive to say. For instance, he might focus on comfort and quality of life for a person without treatment options.
- **Match your language to the patient's words.** It's important to choose words that patients can understand and relate to. Grossman does this by matching his language to the patient's words. For example, he might talk about a "cancerous tumor" with a scientist and a "spot on the colon" with someone unfamiliar with medical terminology.

- **Follow-up.** Patients and their families quickly become overloaded after hearing sad or bad news. When this happens, they are not likely to retain what you are saying. To help people who are reeling from bad news, summarize the most important two or three key points and then bring closure to the conversation. As needed, you might follow this by making plans to talk again at a later time.

When Dealing with Memory Loss or Other Cognitive Challenges

- **Connect new pieces of information to old.** It is much easier to re-member unfamiliar or new information when it is linked to something familiar. Healthcare providers can do this by introducing new informa-tion within a known context. One way is to use a metaphor or analogy. For instance, you might explain an aneurysm by comparing it to a leak-ing garden hose. (Read more in "Metaphors, Similes, and Analogies" starting on page 139.)
- **Chunk information.** Studies show that people can hold on to only about three to five pieces of information at a time before they either lose it or store it in their long-term memory. Healthcare providers can help patients better remember by "chunking" health information into shorter segments. For instance, patients are more likely to succeed at remembering which high-fiber foods to buy if they think in terms of breakfast foods, dinner foods, and then snack items rather than trying to remember all items in a single list.
- **Write down important information.** Most people can remember spoken information better when they have a written (visual) reminder of the conversation. Ideally, patients would take notes during even routine medical appointments. This way, they would have a way to remember all their new data, including weight, height, blood pressure, and any new diagnoses or follow-up instructions. But realistically this is unlikely to happen. Providers can assist by writing a brief summary of what was discussed and giving a copy to the patient.
- **Encourage the use of memory aids.** These can include taping ap-pointments so patients have an audio reminder to listen to at home, or using mnemonics—a word or phrase that uses the first letter of each word in a string of important words (for instance, the U.S. Department of Health and Human Services [2006] uses "DASH" in-stead of "Dietary Approaches to Stop Hypertension" in its publication on lowering blood pressure).
- **Use teach-back to confirm understanding.** Teach-back is a tech-nique in which patients are asked to explain what they've just heard.

It helps by revisiting key concepts throughout appointments and again at the end—providing an opportunity to clarify issues the patient may have missed or found confusing. (Read more in "Confirming Understanding: Teach-Back Technique" starting on page 41.)

Stories from Practice: Cognitive Challenges and Health Literacy

Cognitive challenges vary widely. Some are lifelong, as with intellectual and developmental differences. Other cognitive challenges happen later in life, perhaps due to dementia or brain injury. And as I know from working as a psychiatric occupational therapist, acute and chronic mental illness can also affect concentration, memory, and communication.

To learn more about cognitive challenges and health literacy, I spoke with Joan Guthrie Medlen, MEd, RD, LD, who is a health literacy advocate and author of *The Down Syndrome Nutrition Handbook: A Guide to Promoting Healthy Lifestyles*. Medlen and I share the frustration that there are not many resources looking specifically at this topic. We encourage researchers, clinicians, and other health literacy advocates to help build a knowledge base about effective communication strategies when it comes to health communication and cognition.

Sources: Medlen (2010).

 When we, or those we love and care for, are ill or injured, our emotions can override even the best of communications.

Citations

Medlen JEG. 2006. *The Down Syndrome Nutrition Handbook: A Guide to Promoting Healthy Lifestyles.* Bethesda, MD: Woodbine House.

Medlen JEG. 2010. Telephone interview with author.

Osborne H. 2005, May/June. In Other Words . . . Communicating Bad and Sad News. *On Call.* Available at http://www.healthliteracy.com/bad-sad-news Accessed September 23, 2010.

Osborne H. 2005, October. In Other Words . . . Know When to Speak and When to Listen . . . Communicating With People Who Are Anxious or Angry. *On Call.* Available at http://www.healthliteracy.com/anxious-angry-patients. Accessed January 23, 2011.

Osborne H. 2008, January 10. In Other Words . . . How Memory Affects Health Understanding. *On Call*. Available at http://www.healthliteracy.com/memory Accessed January 23, 2011.

U.S. Department of Health and Human Services. 2006. *Your Guide to Lowering Your Blood Pressure with DASH*. NIH Publication No. 06-4082. Available at http://www.nhlbi.nih.gov/health/public/heart/hbp/dash/new_dash.pdf. Accessed January 23, 2011.

SOURCES TO LEARN MORE

The Centre for Developmental Disability Health Victoria. 2008. *Fact Sheet: Working with People with Intellectual Disabilities in Healthcare Settings*. Available at http://www.cddh.monash.org/assets/documents/working-with-people-with-intellectual-disabilities-in-health-care.pdf. Accessed January 22, 2011. The index page is at http://cddh.monash.org/products-resources.html

Lincoln A, Espejo D, Johnson P, Paasche-Orlow M, Speckman JL, Webber TL, et al. 2008. Limited Literacy and Psychiatric Disorders Among Users of an Urban Safety-Net Hospital's Mental Health Outpatient Clinic. *Journal of Nervous and Mental Disease*. 196(9):687–693.

Osborne H. 2002, September. In Other Words . . . Help Them Talk . . . Communicating with Patients and Families About End-of-Life Decisions. *On Call*. Available at http://www.healthliteracy.com/end-of-life. Accessed January 23, 2011.

Weiss BD, Francis L, Senf JH, Heist K, Hargraves R. 2006. Literacy Education as Treatment for Depression in Patients with Limited Literacy and Depression: A Randomized Controlled Trial. *Journal of General Internal Medicine*. 21(8):823–828.

Know Your Audience: Hearing Loss

STARTING POINTS

Hearing loss ranges from being hard of hearing (mild hearing loss) to being deaf (total hearing loss). People who are deaf from birth often identify themselves as Deaf (with an uppercase "D") to indicate that they are part of a specific cultural and linguistic community. More commonly, people lose hearing as they age. In fact, according to the American Speech-Language-Hearing Association, more than one-half of all people aged 65 and older have some form of hearing loss.

People who are Deaf or hard of hearing need to communicate in ways other than talking and listening. Many Deaf people use sign language. There are a lot of different sign languages, including American Sign Language (ASL). ASL is more than simply using hand gestures to substitute for spoken English. It is a complex language with its own grammar and syntax that makes use of facial expressions, body movements, and hand signs.

Other strategies that people with hearing loss may use include reading lips, communicating in writing, or using assistive listening devices such as hearing aids and telephone amplification systems. Using these methods is not just common courtesy. The 1990 United States Americans with Disabilities Act (ADA) requires that public facilities, including hospitals and health centers, communicate in ways that people with hearing loss can understand.

> **Stories from Practice: Speaking and Listening in a Dental Office**
>
> ---
>
> Here is a story as told to me by someone with hearing loss. Alice, who is hard of hearing, just started going to a new dental office. She lets the staff know that she has a progressive hearing loss and wears a hearing aid. Betty, the dental hygienist, assumes that Alice's hearing aid adequately compensates for her hearing loss and so continues to communicate with Alice as she does with other patients. They speak only briefly before Betty puts on her mask to clean Alice's teeth. This is a problem, however, as Alice can only hear Betty's voice but not distinguish her words.
>
> Six months later, Alice has an appointment with a new hygienist, Cindy. Cindy turns off the radio in the office and sits down to talk with Alice. They discuss what will happen during the cleaning procedure and, together, figure out how to communicate when Cindy wears her mask. Needless to say, Alice feels more positive about this appointment and understands the information that Cindy is communicating.

STRATEGIES, IDEAS, AND SUGGESTIONS

Here are some strategies you might want to try (Osborne 2003):

Determine the preferred method for communicating. Ask Deaf patients and those who are hard of hearing how they prefer to communicate. This may be moving your chair to face patients directly so they can see your lips, communicating in writing, or using an ASL interpreter. Find out also whether patients use assistive listening devices or other types of electronic equipment (more information follows).

Consider the environment. Meet in a quiet space that is free of distracting noises such as air conditioners or overhead pages. Look for a space that has adequate lighting so that the other person can clearly see you when you talk. As appropriate, tap people lightly on their shoulders to get their attention and to orient them to where the sound is coming from. You can convey a sense of welcome by using basic sign language phrases and greetings.

Articulate clearly. Speak distinctly, not necessarily loudly. Shouting is unpleasant and not helpful as it distorts mouth movements and makes lip reading more difficult. Shouting may also interfere with a hearing aid's ability to pick up usable sounds. Instead, use a slower rate of speech, but don't exaggerate pronunciation to the point that you distort individual words.

Facilitate lip reading. People lip-read when they look at someone's mouth and speech-read when they also look at the other person's gestures, expressions, and pantomime actions. Messages are sometimes misinterpreted because pairs of words look alike; for example, "bed" and "men," or "pain" and "main." People who rely on visual cues may have particular difficulty understanding someone who has a mustache or speaks with an accent. To improve understanding, do not cover your mouth, chew gum, or talk at the same time as someone else.

Be aware that written notes don't always work. It is widely assumed that all people with hearing losses benefit from written information. But this is not necessarily so—particularly for those who have been Deaf since birth and, despite normal intelligence, may read only at a fourth- to fifth-grade level. One reason for this lower reading level is that those who have never heard speech cannot "sound out" words—a technique that hearing people commonly use to figure out unfamiliar words. Rather than assume that written notes will help, ask the other person about the best way to communicate.

Utilize electronic devices and equipment. Enhanced technology is opening up a lot of communication options for people with hearing loss. A while ago, TTY (telephone typewriter, a device that allows people with hearing or speech loss to communicate by telephone) was commonly used. Today's options include email, text messaging, and video phones. No doubt, there will be more electronic devices and equipment available in years ahead.

Use ASL interpreters. When communicating with people who use ASL, ask to work with certified or qualified interpreters whose competency is verified according to professional and regulatory standards. Despite good intentions, untrained family members or friends who volunteer to interpret may not be skilled at communicating medical information and may also bring confidentiality and privacy concerns.

With a trained interpreter, start by making sure the patient is comfortable with the interpreter and familiar with the specific sign language being used. (ASL is not the only sign language.) Throughout the session, speak directly to the patient and not the interpreter. Position yourself so that the interpreter sits a little behind you and to the side. This way, the patient can see you and the interpreter in the same visual field. You, in turn, can listen to the interpreter while looking directly at the patient. You can find a database of interpreters for the Deaf at http://www.rid.org. (Read more in "Interpreters and Translations," starting on page 81.)

Confirm understanding. As with all types of health communication, take time to confirm understanding. Whether communicating directly or through an interpreter, ask Deaf and hard-of-hearing patients to tell you, in their own words, their understanding of the topics discussed. If a concept is unclear, rephrase it rather than just repeating it. Confirm understanding throughout your time together, not just when appointments are almost over. (Read more in "Confirm Understanding: Teach-Back Technique," starting on page 41.)

> *People lip-read when they look at someone's mouth and speech-read when they also look at the other person's gestures, expressions, and pantomime actions. Messages are sometimes misinterpreted because pairs of words look alike; for example, "bed" and "men," or "pain" and "main."*

CITATIONS

American Speech-Language-Hearing Association, www.asha.org

Osborne H. 2003. In Other Words . . . Communicating About Health with ASL. *On Call.* 6(6):16–17. Available at http://www.healthliteracy.com/american-sign-language. Accessed July 22, 2010.

U.S. Department of Justice. 1990. *Americans with Disabilities Act of 1990, As Amended.* Available at http://www.ada.gov/pubs/ada.htm. Accessed July 22, 2010.

SOURCES TO LEARN MORE

Barnett S. 1999. Clinical and Cultural Issues in Caring for Deaf People. *Family Medicine.* 31(1):17–22.

Barnett S. 2002. Communication with Deaf and Hard-of-Hearing People: A Guide for Medical Education. *Academic Medicine.* 77(7):694–700.

Barnett S. 2002. Cross-Cultural Communication with Patients Who Use American Sign Language. *Family Medicine.* 34(5):376–382.

D.E.A.F., Inc., http://www.deafinconline.org

Know Your Audience: Literacy

STARTING POINTS

What is literacy? The 2003 U.S. *National Assessment for Adult Literacy (NAAL)* is the most recent and comprehensive measure of adult literacy since the 1992 *National Adult Literacy Survey (NALS)*.

NAAL defines literacy as using "printed and written information to function in society, to achieve one's goals, and to develop one's knowledge and potential." Within this broad definition, there are three types of literacy:

- **Prose literacy.** Needed to understand and use text found in materials like newspapers, magazines, and books.
- **Document literacy.** Required for items such as applications, schedules, forms, maps, graphs, and tables.
- **Quantitative literacy.** Necessary for arithmetic operations such as those found on bank forms and purchase orders.

NAAL *definitions and key findings.* The U.S. Department of Education assessed the literacy level of adults across the United States in 1992 and again in 2003. It did so by asking people to complete a series of word-based tasks. Based on their scores, those tested were determined to be at a below basic, basic, intermediate, or proficient level of literacy. Here is how *NAAL* defines these terms:

- **Below Basic** indicates no more than the most simple and concrete literacy skills.

- **Basic** indicates skills necessary to perform simple and everyday literacy activities.
- **Intermediate** indicates skills necessary to perform moderately challenging literacy activities.
- **Proficient** indicates skills necessary to perform more complex and challenging literacy activities.

Key findings of *NAAL* look at race/ethnicity, age, and educational attainment. Overall, scores show that:

- **Prose literacy:** 14% are at a below basic level; 29% are at a basic level; 44% are at an intermediate level; 13% are at a proficient level.
- **Document literacy:** 12% are at a below basic level: 22% at a basic level; 53% are at an intermediate level; 13% are at a proficient level.
- **Quantitative literacy:** 22% are at a below basic level; 33% are at a basic level; 33% are at an intermediate level; 13% are at a proficient level.

You can find much more data, including state and county estimates of low literacy, at the *NAAL* Web site (http://nces.ed.gov/naal).

Skills that readers need. John Comings, EdD, is an expert on literacy. In a *Health Literacy Out Loud* podcast, he talked about the skills that a reader needs in order to make meaning of written information. These include: (1) print skills, knowing that certain letter combinations have specific sounds; (2) fluency, which includes reading speed and accuracy; (3) vocabulary, knowledge of common, everyday words as well as those more rarely used; and (4) comprehension, integration of all these skills. Readers also need to be able to put these skills into practice as needed for tasks such as completing questionnaires and understanding written directions.

Comings explains that those reading at a below basic literacy level may have physical, mental, or cognitive barriers, such as reading disabilities. They may also, or instead, have limited English skills or be of advanced age. He adds that, on average, literacy skills start to decline when people are 55 years old, and over. Comings says that people reading at a basic literacy level may be undereducated, having dropped out of or barely gotten through high school. They also may lack sufficient reading practice, meaning they do not read often or a lot (Osborne 2010, July 13).

Why literacy matters in health care. People with below basic or basic literacy skills are likely to have difficulty understanding health information as so much of it is communicated in writing. This includes prescription labels, health history forms, self-care instructions, and wellness information.

Stories from Practice: X-Ray to Exit

Here is a story as told to me by a "new reader" (an adult who recently learned to read). Jim is of average intelligence but has dyslexia and can barely read. He went to the doctor for a chronic cough and was told he needed an X-ray. Jim went to a medical center where he hadn't been before and looked for signs saying "X-ray." He didn't see any and was unaware that he needed to instead follow the signs to the "Radiology Department."

The closest word Jim saw to "X-ray" was "Exit." Frustrated and unwilling to let others know that he can barely read, Jim left the medical center and didn't return. Unfortunately, his cough went undiagnosed and untreated.

STRATEGIES, IDEAS, AND SUGGESTIONS

Here are some suggestions to put into practice (Osborne 2010; Comings 2011):

Know about reading difficulties. For many people, literacy problems are a great source of shame. It seldom is advisable to ask a person if he or she can read. Instead, set a tone that is open and feels safe so the person feels more comfortable revealing any reading difficulties.

There is active discussion within the health literacy community about whether routine literacy testing makes sense in clinical situations. Many think that tests like the REALM (Rapid Estimate of Adult Literacy in Medicine) and the TOFHLA (Test of Functional Health Literacy in Adults) are better used for research, not the clinic. I share this point of view.

Instead of formal tests like these, providers may choose to learn about their patient's learning styles and literacy skills by asking open-ended questions. For example, "Do you like to learn by watching TV, listening to the radio, talking with people, or reading?" Indeed, patients with limited literacy skills are apt to select non-reading options.

Another way to get a sense of literacy levels is by noticing "red flags" of reading difficulties. For example, patients with limited reading skills may:

- "Forget" their eyeglasses or complain of headaches each time they are asked to complete paperwork.
- Identify medications by color and shape, not prescription label.
- Have a lot of misspelled words when filling out forms.

- Ask a lot of questions about topics written about in handouts.
- Answer "no" to all health history questions so as to not get more questions.
  (Read more in "Assessing Health Literacy," starting on page 9.)

Use consistent terms and common words. Make it easier for readers to understand by using consistent wording. This includes using the same form of a word, such as "surgery" and not also "surgeries" or "surgical." Refer to items and procedures with the same wording each time, such as "stitch" or "suture." If possible, use common one- and two-syllable words. But, when more complicated words are truly needed, like "chemotherapy" or "bronchodilator," use them and give easy-to-understand examples. When you must use medical jargon or acronyms like "HIPAA" or "GERD," make sure patients know what these terms mean. And try not to use words that sound alike, such as "gait/gate," or have multiple meanings, like "stool" and "dressing." Homonyms like these are especially hard for new or struggling readers to understand. (Read more in "Jargon, Acronyms, and Other Troublesome Words" starting on page 87.)

Select written materials that are sufficiently easy to read. When writing for those who read at a basic literacy level, it is often recommended that materials be written at a fifth- to eighth-grade reading level. When writing for those with below basic literacy skills, materials should be written at a third- to fifth-grade reading level. But writing at these levels is often very hard to do. (Read more in "Assessing Readability with Grade Level Formulas," starting on page 15.)

If all you have are more difficult materials, make it easier for readers by highlighting or circling key points. Encourage readers to look again at these materials when they are relaxed, have sufficient time, or are with others who can help explain unfamiliar words.

Offer non-written options. These include other forms of teaching tools such as pictographs, objects, and videos. You might also consider using assistive technology, such as devices, programs, or Web sites that read text aloud or help people complete forms by offering a choice of answers rather than just blank spaces. Keep in mind that even oral communications should employ vocabulary that most people already know.

Collaborate with new readers and the adult educational system. As Comings and other literacy experts, teachers, and new readers know, an excellent way to improve health understanding is by forming partnerships of healthcare organizations and adult education programs. Such partnerships can not only teach new readers about health but also help healthcare organizations be more "literacy friendly."

 The 2003 U.S. National Assessment for Adult Literacy (NAAL) *defines literacy as the set of skills needed to "use printed and written information to function in society, to achieve one's goals, and to develop one's knowledge and potential."*

CITATIONS

Comings J. 2011. Personal communication.

National Center for Education Statistics. 2003. *National Assessment of Adult Literacy (NAAL).* Available at http://nces.ed.gov/naal. Accessed December 30, 2010.

Osborne H (host). 2010, July 13. Health Literacy from a Literacy Perspective [audio podcast]. *Health Literacy Out Loud Podcast,* no. 41. Available at http://www .healthliteracy.com/hlol-literacy-perspective. Accessed August 16, 2010.

SOURCES TO LEARN MORE

Doak CC, Doak LG, Root JH. 1996. *Teaching Patients with Low Literacy Skills.* 2nd ed. Philadelphia: J. B. Lippincott. Available at http://www.hsph.harvard.edu/ healthliteracy/resources/doak-book/. Accessed April 1, 2011.

Harvard School of Public Health, Health Literacy Studies, www.hsph.harvard.edu/ healthliteracy

Klass P. 2007. When Paper Is The Enemy. *Health Affairs.* 26(2):515–519.

National Adult Education Professional Development Consortium, http://www .naepdc.org/Members/members_home.html. To locate your state office of adult education.

National Adult Literacy Database [Canada], www.nald.ca

National Center for the Study of Adult Learning and Literacy (NCSALL), www .ncsall.net

Osborne H. 2004. In Other Words . . . Healthcare Communication from an Adult Learner's Perspective. *On Call.* Available at http://www.healthliteracy.com/ adult-learner. Accessed August 16, 2010.

Osborne H (host). 2008, October 20. Archie Willard Talks About Struggling to Read [audio podcast]. *Health Literacy Out Loud Podcast,* no. 3. Available at http:// healthliteracy.com/hlol-archie-willard. Accessed August 16, 2010.

U.S. Department of Education, Office of Vocation and Adult Education, http:// www2.ed.gov/about/offices/list/ovae/pi/AdultEd/index.html

Know Your Audience: Older Adults

STARTING POINTS

Adults aged 65 years and older are a significant and ever-increasing percentage of the United States population. Collectively, older adults are a remarkably diverse group, as people in their mid-60s are apt to have far different needs and abilities than those who are two, three, or more decades older. Individually, older adults of course can differ even more.

Despite this diversity, a commonality as people age is that they are increasingly likely to be diagnosed with acute illnesses and chronic conditions. Consequently, older adults and their caretakers (if any) need to learn a lot about health and wellness, treatment and care, and emergency response. But learning this can be a challenge. Reasons include that health information is inherently complex and filled with many new words, concepts, instructions, and devices. Also, older adults may have diseases or take medications that affect their seeing, hearing, alertness, or attention span. Emotional issues, too, can make learning difficult. It is indeed hard for anyone to concentrate when dealing with stresses like selling a home or losing a spouse and close friends.

Stories from Practice: Age-Related Changes Can Affect Health Understanding

Carolyn Ijams Speros, DNSc, FNP-BC, is a nationally recognized expert in nursing and patient education. In a *Health Literacy Out Loud* podcast, she spoke about cognitive and physical changes of aging that can affect health understanding.

Speros said that cognitive challenges can include problems of "mental multitasking," or putting a lot of pieces of information together. There may also be a decline in "fluid intelligence," or the process of reasoning. Speros says that both of these can lead to frustration when older adults try to manage and recall many bits of information from short-term memory. To help, she recommends teaching just three or four key points at one time.

Speros says that visual and auditory changes also impact health understanding. These include changes to the structure of the eye as well as diminished visual acuity. With printed materials, you can help by making sure that the font size is sufficiently large and avoiding colors such as blue that may be hard to see. Auditory changes may affect how well people hear high-pitched sounds, such as female voices. Speros recommends lowering the pitch of your voice somewhat and facing patients directly so they can see, not just hear, what you are saying. Speros adds that there's no benefit in shouting.

Source: Osborne (2010, December 14).

STRATEGIES, IDEAS, AND SUGGESTIONS

Here are some strategies to consider when working with older adults (Osborne 1999; 2001; 2002; 2010, December 14):

Offer a positive and supportive approach. Create "shame-free" learning environments in which older adults can comfortably acknowledge when they do not understand. Let patients who seem confused know they are not the only ones having trouble—that many people find it hard to learn new health information. When possible, offer assistance with filling out paperwork or finding unfamiliar locations.

Create an environment conducive to learning. Make sure that your environment is accessible to people with disabilities and conducive to learning and communication. Here are some ways:

- Post large, readable signs that clearly inform people where they are.
- Provide well-lit rooms, halls, and quiet spaces in which to meet and talk.
- Don't rely just on color to help people navigate the environment, as color-coded arrows may be of no use to people who are color-blind or visually impaired.

Speak in ways people can hear. Speak slowly, clearly, and concisely, and introduce just one new concept at a time. Use everyday language with words that older adults know and are comfortable with. Pay attention as well to nonverbal communication—both yours and the patient's. Throughout your conversation, pause periodically for the patient's questions and to confirm understanding.

Make sure written information is readable. Informally assess the patient's reading skills by paying attention to clues of literacy problems, such as when people repeatedly "forget" their eyeglasses. Rather than ask people if they can read, you might ask how far they went in school—but appreciate that the last grade completed does not necessarily indicate reading ability. In fact, most people read up to five grade levels lower than their last completed year of school. Provide older adults with printed materials that are written in plain language, and have examples and illustrations they can understand and relate to. The best way to know if written materials meet the needs of readers is to ask. (Read more in "Confirming Understanding: Feedback from Interviews, Focus Groups, and Usability Testing," starting on page 35.)

Provide multiple ways for people to learn. Show, not just tell, people about health information. For example, supplement spoken and written information with pictographs and illustrations, CDs and videos, or demonstrations using real objects or simulated models. You can also help older adults learn by sharing stories—yours or theirs—to help them connect with health information in a more personal way.

Help patients participate. Encourage older patients to bring lists of their concerns and questions to appointments. When you meet, discuss a patient's goals and confidence in managing her or his illness. Periodically ask for questions, but be sensitive to the fact that many older adults were brought up to not question medical professionals and may be uncomfortable or unwilling to do so.

Help patients remember. Call patients ahead of time to remind them of appointments and afterward to reinforce instructions and answer unanswered questions. Other ways to help patients remember include sending reminder postcards, suggesting they keep notebooks with personal health information, and recommending pillboxes or other adherence aids. Rather than assuming that people know how to use these aids, demonstrate first, such as by filling a pillbox with a week's worth of medicine. Encourage patients to invite a trusted friend or family member to accompany them to appointments. This way, older adults not only learn in the company of people they find supportive but also have a "second pair of eyes and ears" to reinforce and clarify information after appointments are over.

Verify understanding. Regardless of age, make sure that patients understand the information you are communicating. You can do this with the teach-back technique, asking relevant and specific open-ended questions. For example, you might say, "Some people get dizzy after they take this medicine. If this happens, what will you do?" (Read more in "Confirming Understanding: Teach-Back Technique" starting on page 41.)

 Collectively, older adults are a remarkably diverse group, as people in their mid-60s are apt to have far different needs and abilities than those who are two, three, or more decades older.

CITATIONS

Osborne H. 1999. In Other Words . . Literacy and the Older Adult. *On Call.* Available at http://www.healthliteracy.com/literacy-older-adult. Accessed January 23, 2011.

Osborne H. 2001. In Other Words . . . Mind What You Say . . . Speaking with and Listening to Older Adults. *On Call.* Available at http://www.healthliteracy.com/older-adults. Accessed January 23, 2011.

Osborne H. 2002. In Other Words . . . Making It Work . . . Selecting Healthcare Brochures for Older Adults. *On Call.* Available at http://www.healthliteracy.com/brochures-for-older-adults. Accessed January 23, 2011.

Osborne H (host). 2010, December 14. Communicating About Health with Older Adults [audio podcast]. *Health Literacy Out Loud,* no. 50. Available at http://healthliteracy.com/hlol-older-adults. Accessed January 21, 2011.

Sources to Learn More

AgingStats.gov, Federal Interagency Forum on Aging-Related Statistics, http://www.aoa.gov/Agingstatsdotnet/Main_Site/Default.aspx

Bennett IM, Chen J, Soroui JS, White S. 2009. The Contribution of Health Literacy to Disparities in Self-Rated Health Status and Preventive Health Behaviors in Older Adults. *Annals of Family Medicine.* 7(3):204–211.

Brown H, Prisuta R, Jacobs B, Campbell A. 1996. *Literacy of Older Adults in America.* National Center for Education Statistics. Washington, DC: U.S. Department of Education. Available at http://www.eric.ed.gov/ERICWebPortal/detail?accno=ED402513. Accessed January 21, 2011.

Doak CC, Doak LG, Root JH. 1996. Teaching Patients with Low Literacy Skills. 2nd ed. Philadelphia: J. B. Lippincott. Available at http://www.hsph.harvard.edu/healthliteracy/resources/doak-book/index.html. Accessed December 30, 2010.

Hayes KS. 1998. Randomized Trial of Geragogy-Based Medication Instruction in the Emergency Department. *Nursing Research.* 47(4):211–218.

Helping Older Adults Search for Health Information Online: A Toolkit for Trainers. NIH Senior Health. Available at http://nihseniorhealth.gov/toolkit/toolkit.html Accessed September 24, 2010.

Jansen J, van Weert J, van Dulmen S, Heeren T, Bensing J. 2007. Patient Education About Treatment in Cancer Care: An Overview of the Literature on Older Patients' Needs. *Cancer Nursing.* 30(4):251–260.

Kobylarz FA, Pomidor A, Heath JM. 2006. SPEAK: A Mnemonic Tool for Addressing Health Literacy Concerns in Geriatric Clinical Encounters. *Geriatrics.* 61(7):20–26.

Osborne H (host). 2009, September 8. Age-Related Vision Loss [audio podcast]. *Health Literacy Out Loud Podcast,* no. 21. Available at http://www.healthliteracy.com/hlol-vision-loss. Accessed January 21, 2011.

Pearson M, Wessman J. 1996. Gerogogy in Patient Education. *Home Healthcare Nurse.* 14(8):632–636.

Speros CI. 2005. Health Literacy: Concept Analysis. *Journal of Advanced Nursing.* 50(6):633–640.

Speros CI. 2009. More Than Words: Promoting Health Literacy in Older Adults. *Online Journal of Issues in Nursing.* 14(3):Manuscript 5.

U.S. Department of Health and Human Services, Centers for Medicare and Medicaid Services, by Jeanne McGee of McGee & Evers Consulting. 2010. Part 9: Material for Older Adults. *Toolkit for Making Written Material Clear and Effective.* Available at http://www.cms.gov/WrittenMaterialsToolkit/11_ToolkitPart09.asp Accessed January 21, 2011.

U.S. Department of Health and Human Services. *Quick Guide to Health Literacy and Older Adults.* Available at http://www.health.gov/communication/literacy/olderadults/literacy.htm. Accessed August 5, 2010.

Zurakowski T, Taylor M, Bradway C. 2006. Effective Teaching Strategies for the Older Adult with Urologic Concerns. *Urologic Nursing.* 26(5):355–360.

Know Your Audience: Vision Problems

STARTING POINTS

According to the American Foundation for the Blind, people with visual problems may have trouble seeing, even when wearing glasses or contact lenses, or are blind and cannot see at all. The foundation cites a national study showing that more than 25 million adults in the United States report experiencing significant vision loss.

Health facilities are required to accommodate the needs of people with vision problems. The 1990 Americans with Disabilities Act mandates that public facilities (like hospitals and health centers) provide reasonable accommodations for people who are blind or visually impaired. These facilities must provide information in large print, audiotape, Braille formats, or have someone available to read information aloud.

STRATEGIES, IDEAS, AND SUGGESTIONS

Here are some suggestions to consider (Osborne 2000; 2009):

Ask if the person wants assistance. The amount of assistance a person with vision loss desires depends on the situation and his or her comfort in asking. Ask if she or he wants help, and if so, find out how you can best be of assistance. The person may want descriptive or directional information, such as identifying where objects are located within a room, or explaining

> ### Stories from Practice: Age-Related Vision Loss
>
> Cynthia Stuen, PhD, MSW, is Senior Vice President and Chief Professional Affairs Officer at Lighthouse International. She talked about age-related vision loss in a *Health Literacy Out Loud* podcast.
>
> Stuen says that everyone's vision changes with age. Some changes are normal, such as a condition called presbyopia, in which the lens of the eye becomes less elastic, making it harder to focus. It gets harder to differentiate between colors, and one needs more light. Other age-related vision problems are due to medical conditions. These may affect the central field of vision (such as from macular degeneration), peripheral or side vision (glaucoma), or overall vision (such as from diabetic retinopathy or cataracts).
>
> It is not always easy to know if someone has age-related vision loss. Whether due to the slow rate of visual changes, denial, or fear, older adults may not realize the extent of their visual problems. Stuen offers some signs to look for that indicate the person may be having difficulty with vision:
>
> - Is the person making direct eye contact with you? If not, perhaps he or she is using peripheral, rather than central, vision.
> - Does the person trip a lot or frequently bump into objects? Perhaps he or she has trouble seeing environmental impediments.
> - Has the person stopped participating in usual activities? Maybe a lifelong bridge player is finding reasons not to play because he or she cannot see the cards.
>
> *Source:* Osborne (2009, September 8).

any unusual sounds or noises. The person may also ask to take your elbow and walk alongside you.

Some people, however, may choose not to reveal their blindness, especially at initial meetings. As a matter of practice you should ask all patients, "Would you like that information in any other format?" Talk with patients about function, rather than vision. Ask, for example, "How can I help you?" rather than "How much can you see?" The amount of assistance a person desires depends on the situation and his or her comfort in asking.

Introduce yourself and others. Identify yourself by name when you enter a room where there is a person who is blind or has significant vision loss. When a person comes into the room, introduce yourself and everyone else who is present. When someone leaves the room, communicate this to the person with impaired vision.

Use everyday words. Give clear, specific information and use common words, not medical jargon. Don't be afraid to use verbs such as "see" and "look"; they are a part of everyday speech.

Provide clear directions. Be specific and descriptive. When you refer a patient to a new facility, make sure that person is comfortable going to an unfamiliar location. One way you can help is by giving detailed directions that make use of landmarks. Be sure, however, you talk about "left" and "right" from the other person's perspective, not your own.

Use design to help people with limited vision see written materials.

- Use a simple font and avoid italics or other stylized or decorative lettering.
- Use at least a 12-point type for "regular" readers. For those with limited vision, increase the print size to 16 to 18 points, which is the standard for large print.
- Have a high contrast between the color of the foreground and background. Black lettering on white, yellow, or other light-colored paper provides good contrast.
- Use matte rather than glossy paper to reduce glare.
- Have margins that are at least an inch wide, and increase line spacing from single space to at least one and a half spaces.
- When writing by hand, write in large-sized letters using thick, felt-tip markers.
- Use print or block lettering rather than script, and avoid writing or typing in all capital letters because this format is difficult to read (Arditi 2002).

Choose contrasting colors. People with partial sight or color deficiencies may have trouble distinguishing between certain color combinations. Compensate for these difficulties by choosing colors that are drastically different in terms of their tone (basic color), lightness (how much light is reflected), and saturation (the intensity of color) (Arditi 2002).

Stuen recommends contrasting colors that are opposite each other on the color wheel, such as yellow and violet. Of course, white and black work well too. When deciding whether to have dark lettering on a light background (as is common) or light print on dark background, there is no firm rule. What matters most is that the contrast is really good and can be read, says Stuen.

Talk with patients about nonvisual sensory cues. For example, when teaching a person how to recognize signs of a wound infection, include the warning symptoms of oozing, swelling, tenderness, smell, and sensation of heat in addition to redness. As well, help patients learn nonvisual ways to accomplish tasks. For example, if a person is having difficulty seeing the numbers on a thermometer—even with a magnifier—let him or her know that a talking thermometer is available.

Signage. Use both Braille and large print to identify offices, room numbers, departments, building directories, elevator call buttons, and elevator door jambs (panels by the door that indicate the floor number). Make sure printed signs have sufficient contrast between foreground and background and that the background of the sign contrasts with the wall color.

Offer referrals, tools, and resources.

- If you are working with someone who may have low vision, consider making a referral to eye care doctors who specialize in low vision and vision rehabilitation.
- Let the other person know about helpful aids such as magnifiers, telescopic lenses, and prismatic lenses that may be prescribed.
- Maintain a library of high-quality non-print patient education materials. These can include Books On Tape® and podcasts. When using visuals, make sure the narration adequately describes the images.

Find creative solutions. People who are visually impaired may have trouble distinguishing one medication from another because pill bottles are often identical in shape and size. One way people with vision problems can tell the two medications apart is by putting one rubber band (or piece of tape) on the first bottle and two rubber bands (or pieces of tape) on the second. Another way is by asking pharmacists to put the different medications in two differently shaped containers. In addition, people with vision problems might keep one medication in the bedroom and another in the kitchen to keep track of which is which.

Make sure online materials are accessible.

- When designing or updating Web sites, follow the guidelines for accessibility as described in W3C: Web Accessibility Initiative. To learn more, go to http://www.w3.org/WAI/.
- Know about tools that allow people with low vision to access online information. An example is "LowBrowse" from Lighthouse International. This free add-on extension to the Firefox Web browser allows people to set the formats that meet their needs as low vision users. To learn more, go to http://www.lighthouse.org/services-and-assistance/computers-and-technology/computer/lowbrowse/.

 Give clear, specific information and use common words, not medical jargon. Don't be afraid to use verbs such as "see" and "look"; they are a part of everyday speech.

CITATIONS

American Foundation for the Blind. 2010. *Facts and Figures on Adults with Vision Loss.* Available at http://www.afb.org/Section.asp?SectionID=15&TopicID=413&DocumentID=4900. Accessed September 18, 2010.

Arditi A. n.d. *Effective Color Contrast: Designing for People with Partial Sight and Color Deficiencies.* Lighthouse International. http://www.lighthouse.org/accessibility/design/accessible-print-design/effective-color-contrast. Accessed September 18, 2010.

Arditi A. n.d. *Making Text Legible: Designing for People with Partial Sight. Lighthouse International.* Available at http://www.lighthouse.org/accessibility/design/accessible-print-design/making-text-legible. Accessed September 18, 2010.

Osborne H. 2000, October. In Other Words . . . When Vision Is an Issue . . . Communicating with Patients Who Are Visually Impaired. *On Call.* http://www.healthliteracy.com/visually-impaired. Accessed September 18, 2010.

Osborne H (host). 2009, September 8. Age-Related Vision Loss [audio podcast]. *Health Literacy Out Loud,* no. 21. Available at http://healthliteracy.com/hlol-vision-loss. Accessed September 18, 2010.

SOURCES TO LEARN MORE

American Foundation for the Blind. 2010. *Guidelines for Prescription Labeling and Consumer Medication Information for People with Vision Loss.* Available at http://www.afb.org/Section.asp?SectionID=3&TopicID=329&DocumentID=4064 Accessed August 6, 2010.

Harrison TC, Mackert M, Watkins C. 2010. A Quantitative Analysis of Health Literacy Issues Among Women with Visual Impairments. *Research in Gerontological Nursing.* 3(1):49–60.

Lighthouse International, www.lighthouse.org

National Eye Institute, http://www.nei.nih.gov

National Federation of the Blind, www.nfb.org

U.S. Department of Justice. 1990. *Americans with Disabilities Act of 1990, As Amended.* Available at http://www.ada.gov/. Accessed September 18, 2010.

Listening and Speaking

STARTING POINTS

Just because listening and speaking happen a lot doesn't mean that this form of communication is always easy or effective. For instance, speaking can be hard when providers are rushed, explain the same concepts over and over again, or assume that patients understand everything being said. For patients, listening can be hard because of complicated concepts like risks and benefits, abstract ideas such as wellness, and multisyllabic terms that may sound to patients like a foreign language. Despite these many challenges, providers have a responsibility to communicate health information in ways that patients and their families or caregivers can understand.

STRATEGIES, IDEAS, AND SUGGESTIONS

Here are some ideas you might use in practice (Osborne 2000, March; 2006, January/February; 2008, January):

Try to find a private, quiet, well-lit place in which to talk. The space you meet in is almost as important as the topics you discuss. If a separate room is not available, at least pull curtains or move chairs to create a sense of privacy. (Read more in "Environment of Care," starting on page 57.)

Develop rapport. Set a positive tone by beginning conversations with a smile and warm handshake. Introduce yourself by the name you wish to be called and, in turn, ask patients how they prefer to be addressed. Meet patients at eye level; sit down if they are seated or in bed. Often, you can build rapport by first chatting about nonmedical matters such as the weather or current events. Make sure the person you are talking with is not so distracted or uncomfortable that meaningful conversation is impossible.

Give patients your undivided attention. You can do this by encouraging patients to fully state their thoughts by saying "that's interesting," or "please tell me more." Make sure not to interrupt and, instead, make a note to yourself of issues to revisit when the patient stops talking.

Choose your words carefully. Health care has its own vocabulary. For example, medical jargon like "dressing" has nothing to do with clothing, salads, or turkeys. Terms like "formulary" and acronyms or initialisms (new "words" made up from longer phrases) such as "ADL" and "HIPAA" may be unknown to patients. And patients can get understandably confused when health professionals interchange words like "hypertension" and "high blood pressure."

When you truly need a word that patients don't already know, explain it and give an example. For instance, say "ADLs—activities of daily living, like getting dressed or eating." Often, you can take cues from patients about which words to use. For example, if they say "sugar" rather than "diabetes," you should feel comfortable doing the same so long as you make clear that it is more commonly called diabetes.

Pay attention to tone of voice, pacing (the speed at which you speak), and sighs. Nonverbal utterances like these can be as expressive as words. Talking quickly and loudly may convey impatience, while a more relaxed and quiet tone can indicate caring and concern. When healthcare providers make eye contact and smile, patients likely get a sense of caring and compassion. But when providers look away or scowl, patients may instead feel that providers are unfriendly or even hostile.

Confirm understanding. Use the teach-back technique to make sure that you and your patients truly understand each other. Start by putting responsibility on yourself (where it rightfully belongs) by saying something along the lines of, "Let me see if I've made myself clear." Then ask relevant and specific open-ended questions like, "Some parents wonder when to call our office. If your child's fever goes over 102 degrees, what will you do?" Or, "What will you tell your friends about this illness?" And, after talking about the dosage for a new liquid medication, you might say, "Show me which sized spoon you will use to take this medicine."

Stories from Practice: The Power of Pausing

Donald Rubin, PhD, is a professor and researcher whose work focuses on assessment, training, and analysis of oral communication, including "listenability." In a *Health Literacy Out Loud* podcast, he spoke about interactive health literacy and oral communication.

Rubin says that silent pauses can be powerful tools when eliciting information. Just as nature abhors a vacuum, he says that conversations abhor silence. "We all have a natural inclination to want to fill that space when we're face to face with somebody." He says that a pause over two seconds is a pretty noticeable. And a pause of 10 seconds can be uncomfortable.

"If a physician or any kind of health care provider is interested in eliciting information from a patient or consumer, imposing those kinds of silent pauses is very powerful. It's probably even more powerful than asking direct questions. A lot of times, patients are not very well prepared to answer questions. They may answer them in very vague ways. When they're confronted with silence, they will open up and do whatever they need to fill that silence," says Rubin.

Source: Osborne (2010, April 13).

Likewise, make sure you understand correctly. Periodically stop and repeat back what you hear patients say. For instance, "I hear you say that you have a lot of shoulder pain. Does this keep you from carrying grocery bags into the house?" This way you not only confirm that you "get it" but also demonstrate that you are listening and paying attention. (Read more in "Confirming Understanding: Teach-Back Technique," starting on page 41.)

Ensure clarity during telephone conversations. In today's busy and wired world, a lot of health communication takes place over the telephone. This includes: one-to-one conversations between patients and providers; conference calls with interpreters, families, or specialists far away; "hotlines" and other crisis services; telephone triage and call centers where health professionals assess a patient's need for care; and recorded messages that you leave for others or they leave for you.

While there are many advantages, especially in terms of access and efficiency, of talking by phone, there are also some drawbacks, as there are no visual cues to confirm understanding. Suzanne O'Connor, RN, MS, suggests some ways to use the phone to an advantage (Osborne 2000.)

- **Have help in your voice.** Set a pleasant tone in order to help the person at the other end of the conversation absorb information. Be as positive as possible, saying "I will" and "I can," rather than "I won't" and "I can't." When you must say "no," state why and offer alternatives.
- **When the caller is cheerful or friendly, respond in a similar fashion.** If the other person is sad or disappointed, be empathetic and acknowledge these feelings. And when the caller is angry or agitated, stay calm and try to defuse the situation.
- **Take responsibility for the direction of the conversation.** Redirect talkative callers. For example, you can say, "I hear your concern about . . . I'd like to help and wonder if you called for an appointment."
- **Choose your words carefully.** Since the phone is auditory only, make sure your words are easy for others to understand. As a rule, this means using common one- and two-syllable words, like saying "doctor" instead of "physician." It also means defining new or complicated terms, such as "durable medical equipment."
- **Set ground rules and clear expectations for conference calls.** Begin by designating a leader who is responsible for the call. The leader should give rules, such as to identify yourself each time you speak, and put the call on mute if you're in a noisy environment. Then the leader should invite all participants to briefly introduce themselves. Throughout the call, the leader should make sure that everyone who wants to speak has the opportunity to do so. At the end of the call, the leader should summarize key points, ask for questions and clarification, and conclude by talking about next steps.
- **Recording messages.** When you leave a message on someone else's machine, speak slowly and clearly. Give your name and phone number at the beginning and again at the end; this way the other person hears twice how to reach you. It is also helpful to leave best times to return your call so as to avoid needless rounds of "telephone tag." Another tip is to stand up when recording voice messages. I've learned from experience that you're likely to sound much more energetic this way.
- **Confirm understanding.** In one-to-one conversations as well as on conference calls, stop periodically and confirm that all parties understand one another. Near the end of the call, summarize what you talked about and the actions everyone agrees to take. After the call, you may want to send a letter or brochure with additional resources and ways for people to learn more.

Make use of new technologies. There are lots of interesting opportunities ahead for communicating with new, or variations on old, technologies, including conference calls, video conferencing, and Skype, to name just a few. Suzanne O'Connor anticipates that telephonic modes of communication like these will become more utilized in the future.

 Nonverbal utterances can be as expressive as words. Talking quickly and loud may convey impatience, while a more relaxed and quiet tone can indicate caring and concern.

CITATIONS

Osborne H. 2000, March. In Other Words . . . Don't Just Stand There, Answer. *On Call.* Available at http://healthliteracy.com/telephone. Accessed January 26, 2011.

Osborne H. 2006, January/February. In Other Words . . . Actions Can Speak as Clearly as Words. *On Call.* Available at http://www.healthliteracy.com/actions Accessed January 25, 2011.

Osborne H. 2008, January 31. In Other Words . . . Actively Listening for What Patients Do Not Say. *On Call.* Available at http://www.healthliteracy.com/ active-listening. Accessed January 25, 2011.

Osborne H (host). 2010, April 13. Talking About Interactive Health Literacy and Oral Communication [audio podcast]. *Health Literacy Out Loud,* no. 35. Available at http://www.healthliteracy.com/hlol-oral-communication Accessed January 26, 2011.

SOURCES TO LEARN MORE

Hydén LC, Mishler EG. 1999. Language and Medicine. *Annual Review of Applied Linguistics.* 19:174–192.

Kelly N. 2008. The Voice on the Other End of the Phone. *Health Affairs.* 27(6): 1701–1706. Available at http://content.healthaffairs.org/content/27/6/1701 .full. Accessed January 26, 2011.

National Literacy and Health Program, Canadian Public Health Association. 1999. *Easy Does It! Plain Language and Clear Verbal Communication.* Ontario, Canada: Canadian Public Health Association. Available at http://www.cpha.ca/uploads/ portals/h-l/easy_does_it_e.pdf. Accessed January 26, 2011.

Osborne H. 2003, May. In Other Words . . . Opening the Interactive Communication Loop. *On Call.* Available at http://www.healthliteracy.com/ interactive-communication-loop. Accessed January 25, 2011.

Rubin DL, Hafer T, Arata K. 2000. Reading and Listening to Oral-Based Versus Literate-Based Discourse. *Communication Education.* 49(2):121–134.

Schillinger D, Piette J, Grumbach K, Wang F, Wilson C, Daher C, et al. 2003. Closing the Loop: Physician Communication with Diabetic Patients Who Have Low Health Literacy. *Archives of Internal Medicine.* 163(1):83–90.

Metaphors, Similes, and Analogies

STARTING POINTS

Metaphors, similes, and analogies are figures of speech used to help people understand unfamiliar words and concepts. They do so by comparing new information to that which people already know. While there are important distinctions among the three forms of speech, for sake of simplicity in this chapter I'll use the overall term "metaphor."

STRATEGIES, IDEAS, AND SUGGESTIONS

Here are ways to put metaphors into practice (Osborne 2003, January; 2003, May):

Determine when to use a metaphor. Some healthcare concepts are straightforward and a simple explanation is sufficient. Save metaphors for those times when you are teaching something that is unfamiliar or hard to understand. For example, you might use a metaphor to explain a new diagnosis like congestive heart failure but not for a well-understood condition like the common cold.

Use words, terms, and examples that people know. To be effective, the person you are speaking with needs to know what your analog (example) means. For instance, saying "getting a vaccination is like installing antivirus software" may have meaning to someone familiar with computers. But if the person prefers camping to computing, you might instead say, "getting a vaccine is like putting on bug spray before going in the woods."

Stories from Practice: Examples of Metaphors

Here are some examples of metaphors that answer the question, "Why don't we use antibiotics for colds, acute bronchitis, and other viral illnesses?"

- "You don't use bug spray to kill weeds in your lawn."
- "Using antibiotics for viruses is like using a large net to catch minnows. They just go through the holes."
- "Using antibiotics for viruses is like putting gas in your gas tank if your battery is dead."
- "Treating a cold with antibiotics is like using an umbrella to stay warm in winter. It just doesn't work, and when it starts to rain, your umbrella might be worn out."

Source: The Altoona List of Medical Analogies, available at http://www.altoonafp.org/analogies

---

Explain the metaphor. Metaphors by themselves are seldom sufficient. After you use one, follow up with a fuller explanation. If you say "an aneurysm is like a bulge in a garden hose," explain how these concepts are alike by saying, "The bigger the bulge, the thinner the wall and the more likely it will burst." Acknowledge limitations of your metaphor, as well. In this instance you might say how aneurysms happen only in certain parts of the body, while garden hoses can get bulges almost everywhere.

Move beyond the metaphor. After you confirm that a patient understands the metaphor, transition to the correct medical terminology. In the example above about an aneurysm, this means teaching important terms like "aortic aneurysm" and "cerebral aneurysm."

Confirm understanding. Metaphors aren't always obvious, nor are they necessarily understood in the way you intend. Sometimes they add to confusion. A physician was explaining to his patient that her heart is "like a pump." He assumed that since the patient lived in a rural area, she would certainly understand the metaphor. While the patient smiled and nodded politely, it wasn't until several visits later that she told her doctor that she had no idea how pumps work. Knowing this, the physician explained her cardiac condition in another way. As with all forms of health communication, make sure that patients truly understand.

 Some healthcare concepts are straightforward and a simple explanation is sufficient. Save metaphors for those times when you are teaching something that is unfamiliar or hard to understand.

CITATIONS

Osborne H. 2003, January. In Other Words . . . It's Like What You Already Know . . . Using Analogies to Help Patients Understand. *On Call*. Available at http://www .healthliteracy.com/analogies. Accessed January 26, 2011.

Osborne H. 2003, May. In Other Words . . . Opening the Interactive Communication Loop. *On Call*. Available at http://www.healthliteracy.com/ interactive-communication-loop. Accessed January 26, 2011.

SOURCES TO LEARN MORE

Clark B. 2011. Metaphor, Simile and Analogy: What's the Difference? [blog]. *Copyblogger*. Available at http://www.copyblogger.com/metaphor-simile-and-analogy-what's-the-difference/. Accessed April 15, 2011.

Jones P, Jones S, Stone D. 2007. Accuracy of Comparing Bone Quality to Chocolate Bars for Patient Information Purposes: Observational Study. *British Medical Journal*. 335:1285–1287.

Lakoff G, Johnson M. 1980. *Metaphors We Live By*. Chicago: University of Chicago Press.

Pink DH. 2006. *A Whole New Mind: Why Right-Brainers Will Rule the Future*. New York: Riverhead Books.

Numeracy

To understand most health information, people need a working knowledge of numbers. This is needed for tasks such as making sense of risk data, selecting healthy foods by reading nutrition labels, estimating costs and figuring budgets, and rating satisfaction or pain on scales from 1 to 10. Numbers-based tasks like these are often referred to as "health numeracy."

What is health numeracy? Golbeck, Ahlers-Schmidt, Paschal, and Dismuke (2005) define health numeracy as "the degree to which individuals have the capacity to access, process, interpret, communicate, and act on numerical, quantitative, graphical, biostatistics, and probabilistic health information needed to make effective health decisions." He categorizes health numeracy skills as:

- **Basic.** This includes skills needed to identify numbers and make sense of quantitative data. These are needed for tasks such as counting pills or knowing the time and date of appointments.
- **Computational.** This includes skills to count, quantify, compute, and manipulate numbers. An example is totaling the number of carbohydrates from a nutrition label.
- **Analytical.** These skills are needed to understand inference, estimation, proportion, percentage, and other high-level concepts. Examples include determining whether cholesterol numbers are within normal range, understanding basic graphs, and comparing insurance benefits.

- **Statistical.** These skills are needed to critically analyze quantitative information to comprehend concepts such as risk and randomization or "blind" studies (Golbeck et al. 2005).

Who has problems with numbers? Nearly all health numeracy studies conclude that the vast majority of the lay public struggle to understand and use numbers. In 2003, the U.S. Department of Education, National Center for Educational Statistics looked at quantitative literacy (needed for calculations and other numeric tasks) as a subset of overall literacy skills. Findings show that:

- 22% of the adults in the United States have below basic quantitative skills
- 33% of the same population has basic quantitative skills
- 33% has intermediate quantitative skills
- 13% has proficient quantitative skills

Some subsets in the populations have even greater difficulty. For example, in this study 71% of older adults (aged 65 and over) scored at a basic or below level of quantitative skills. And 89% of those with less than or some high school education were found to have only basic or below quantitative skills (U.S. Department of Education, National Center for Educational Statistics 2003). (Read more in "Know Your Audience: Literacy" starting on page 115.)

STRATEGIES, IDEAS, AND SUGGESTIONS

Here are some helpful strategies (Osborne 2004; 2007; 2010):

Know why are you using numbers. What message are you trying to convey? Are numbers essential to making this point? If so, be mindful as to your goal, such as using numbers to compare treatment options, encourage certain behaviors, or convey feelings of concern or relief.

Help people make meaning of numbers. For instance, if your patient's cholesterol test came back with a level of 220, help her determine if this is a good result, or bad. One way to do so is by giving additional information such as high and low parameters or what her cholesterol level was last year.

Help people measure correctly. Here are some ways:

- Mark how high to fill a drinking cup. Or use a divided plate to show proper proportions of vegetables, fruits, protein, and grains. The United States Department of Agriculture does just that with its food icon, MyPlate. This visual is available at http://www.choosemyplate.gov/

- Compare quantity to known amounts, such as "4 ounces of meat is about the size of a deck of playing cards."
- Use familiar measurement units such as ounces or grams, cups or liters.
- Demonstrate fractions. Some people may figure that a bigger number always means more. But that is not the case when it comes to fractions. Make it clear by showing pictures such as of a cup that is ⅓ full alongside a cup that is ½ full.

Stories from Practice: Why People Have Trouble with Numbers

Andrea Apter, MD, MA, MSc, is a practicing physician and professor of medicine at the University of Pennsylvania, specializing in the treatment of patients with asthma. She also was a math teacher. In a *Health Literacy Out Loud* podcast, Dr. Apter spoke about why people struggle so much with numbers. She said it can relate to the anxiety of being a patient or be due to a person's math education. She adds that problems with numbers do not necessarily relate to overall intelligence. Dr. Apter shares examples of number-based problems she sees in practice:

- *Figuring out measurements.* "I noticed that if patients were asked to take 30 milligrams of prednisone and given 5-milligram pills, it was very difficult for many people to figure out how many pills they had to take."
- *Reading and tracking numbers.* "As an asthma specialist, we sometimes give patients peak flow meters. These meters may be hard for people to read. In addition, we sometimes ask them to track their readings and put them on a line chart. That may be hard for patients."
- *Understanding risk and other mathematic concepts.* "If a doctor says to a patient, 'If you lose 5 percent of your weight, your blood pressure will be much better and your risk of stroke will be reduced,' in that sentence there are several mathematical concepts. The doctor said '5 percent' instead of saying how many pounds, which might be a simpler concept. Then the doctor said, 'Your risk of dying from a stroke might be reduced.' Risk is a probability."

Source: Osborne (2010, May 25).

Make calculations easier. Sometimes people need to perform calculations such as adding the number of fat grams or dividing a recipe in half. If you are meeting in person, sit alongside each other and do calculations together. In writing, line up calculations, making clear how to handle decimals, such as:

$$\begin{array}{r} 101 \\ 100.2 \\ \underline{+102} \end{array}$$

Give context for number-based concepts. Health information is filled with number-based concepts, including risks, benefits, frequency, and probability. Here are some ways to make such concepts easier to understand:

- Appreciate that while clinicians and scientists may talk in terms of populations (such as "2,753 out of 10,000 people will . . . ") many patients are much more interested in "What will happen to me?"
- Make clear what the risk is about. Talk with the patient about whether this risk is for getting diagnosed with this condition or dying of it.
- When possible, state risk as absolute (a new drug reduces a person's risk from 2 out of 10 to 1 out of 10), not relative (the new drug reduces a person's risk by 50 percent).
- As indicated, frame results as positive (95 percent of patients improve), not negative (5 percent of patients do not improve or get worse).
- Compare unfamiliar concepts to something known. For example, "You can lift up to 5 pounds—about the same weight as a bag of flour." Or "A newborn's tummy is about the size of a . . . "

Recognize that words and symbols sometimes serve as shorthand for numbers and calculations. Informed consent forms, for example, often include terms like "common," "uncommon," and "rare." Here are ways to help:

- To clarify important concepts, use both numbers and words, such as, "A common risk affects at least 4 out of 10 people."
- Avoid vague words that are open to interpretation, such as "adequate," "moderate," and "some."
- Be sensitive to words with multiple meanings. This includes the word "and," which can be meant as "to add" or "also."
- Know that not everyone understands mathematic symbols. These include: $<$, $>$, and $+/-$.
- Be willing to bend the rules. Really, it's often okay to write "5" rather than "five." Or "almost half" rather than "48 percent."

Use charts, graphs, and other visual tools. They include:

- Pie charts to show proportion
- Bar graphs to make comparisons
- Line graphs that communicate trends
- Scatter plots that show variability

You might also include pictures, such as of sun-up and sun-down, to show time of day. Or illustrations to compare measurements, such as two thermometers—one showing a normal temperature and the other a high fever.

Confirm understanding. Make sure patients truly understand numbers and data. You might, for example, ask patients to tell you how they will explain number-based information to a friend or family member. And make sure you truly understand as well. Just because you are a health professional does not make you immune from number trouble.

Stories from Practice: Making an Informed Choice Based on Numbers

Maybe you're like me and of that age when your body parts don't always work the way you want. Several years ago, I was diagnosed with something serious, but treatable. Dr. Tabesh was one of my many medical specialists.

Like most patients and providers, Dr. Tabesh and I talked a lot about medication. She said that there are two very different classes of drugs for women with my health history. She discussed them both and asked me to make an informed choice. To explain the implications, Dr. Tabesh presented detailed data about numbers needed to treat, absolute risk, relative risk, and five-year outcomes.

What I hadn't told her before was that I don't "do" numbers, at least not very well. Luckily, she noticed the blank look on my face and then gestured what these numbers mean: "Here's how much this new drug could help"—holding one hand high. "Here's the risk if you take it"—gesturing low with her other hand.

I'm a visual person. Thanks to her gesture, I "got" what Dr. Tabesh was talking about and made an informed medication choice. What's so special about this story? Nothing, and that's why it's important. Imagine what health care would be like if all providers explained numbers as clearly as Dr. Tabesh.

Make sure you truly understand numbers as well. Just because you are a health professional does not make you immune from number trouble.

CITATIONS

Golbeck AL, Ahlers-Schmidt CR, Paschal AM, Dismuke SE. 2005. A Definition and Operational Framework for Health Numeracy. *American Journal of Preventative Medicine.* 29(4):375–376.

Osborne H. 2004, June/July. In Other Words . . . Working with Numbers. *On Call.* Available at http://www.healthliteracy.com/working-with-numbers. Accessed July 18, 2010.

Osborne H. 2007, September 19. In Other Words . . . Health Numeracy: How Do Patients Handle the Concept of Quantity When It Relates to Their Health? *On Call.* Available at http://www.healthliteracy.com/health-numeracy. Accessed July 18, 2010.

Osborne H (host). 2010, May 25. Health Numeracy: Helping Patients Understand Numeric Concepts [audio podcast]. *Health Literacy Out Loud,* no. 38. Available at http://healthliteracy.com/hlol-numeric-concepts. Accessed January 27, 2011.

U.S. Department of Education, National Center for Educational Statistics. 2003. *National Assessment of Adult Literacy.* Available at http://nces.ed.gov/naal

SOURCES TO LEARN MORE

Agency for Healthcare Research and Quality. 2008. *How to Create a Pill Card.* AHRQ Publication No. 08-M016. Available at http://www.ahrq.gov/qual/pillcard/pillcard.htm. Accessed July 17, 2010.

Apter AJ, Cheng J, Small D, Bennett IM, Albert C, Fein DG, et al. 2009. Asthma Numeracy Skill and Health Literacy. *Journal of Asthma.* 43(9): 705–710.

Apter AJ, Paasche-Orlow MK, Remillard JT, Bennett IM, Ben-Joseph EP, Batista RM, et al. 2008. Numeracy and Communication with Patients: They Are Counting on Us. *Journal of General Internal Medicine.* 23(12): 2117–2124.

Apter AJ, Wang X, Bogen D, Benett IM, Jennings RM, Garcia L, et al. 2009. Linking Numeracy and Asthma-Related Quality of Life. *Patient Education and Counseling.* 75(3):386–391.

Best J. 2001. *Damned Lies and Statistics: Untangling Numbers from the Media, Politicians, and Activists.* Berkeley: University of California Press.

Brown SM, Culver JO, Osann KE, Macdonald DJ, Sand S, Thornton AA, et al. 2011. Health Literacy, Numeracy, and Interpretation of Graphical Breast Cancer Risk Estimates. *Patient Education and Counseling.* 83(1):92–98.

Department of Health (United Kingdom). 1997. *Communicating About Risks to Public Health: Pointers to Good Practice.* Available at http://www.dh.gov.uk/en/Publicationsandstatistics/Publications/PublicationsPolicyAndGuidance/DH_4006604. Accessed January 27, 2011.

Donelle L, Arocha JF, Hoffman-Goetz L. 2008. Health Literacy and Numeracy: Key Factors in Cancer Risk Comprehension. *Chronic Diseases in Canada.* 29(1):1–8.

Edwards A, Elwyn G, Mulley A. 2002. Explaining Risks: Turning Numerical Data into Meaningful Pictures. *British Medical Journal.* 324:827–830.

Fagerlin A, Ubel PA, Smith DM, Zikmund-Fisher BJ. 2007. Making Numbers Matter: Present and Future Research in Risk Communication. *American Journal of Health Behavior.* 31(Supp):S47–S56.

Gigerenzer G, Edwards A. 2003. Simple Tools for Understanding Risks: From Innumeracy to Insight. *British Medical Journal.* 327(7417):741.

Ginsburg L, Manly M, Schmitt MJ. 2006. *The Components of Numeracy.* Cambridge, MA: National Center for the Study of Adult Learning and Literacy. Available at http://www.ncsall.net/fileadmin/resources/research/op_numeracy.pdf. Accessed July 17, 2010.

Hill LH. 2008. The Role of Visuals in Communicating Health Information to Low Literate Adults. *Focus on Basics: Connecting Research and Practice.* 9(B):40–46.

Huizinga MM, Beech BM, Cavanaugh KL, Elasy TA, Rothman RL. 2008. Low Numeracy Skills Are Associated with Higher BMI. *Obesity.* 16(8):1966–1968.

Nielsen J. 2007. Show Numbers as Numerals When Writing for Online Readers. *Jakob Nielsen's Alertbox.* Available at http://www.useit.com/alertbox/writing-numbers.html. Accessed July 17, 2010.

Lipkus IM, Hollands JG. 1999. The Visual Communication of Risk. *Journal of the National Cancer Institute. Monographs.* (25):149–163.

Osborne H. (host). 2011, April 5. Helping Others Understand Health Messages [audio podcast]. *Health Literacy Out Loud,* no. 56. Available at http://healthliteracy.com/hlol-health-messages. Accessed April 8, 2011.

Paling J. 2006. *Helping Patients Understand Risks: 7 Simple Strategies for Successful Communication.* Gainesville, FL: The Risk Communication Institute.

Peters E, Hibbard J, Slovic P, Dieckmann N. 2007. Numeracy Skill and the Communication, Comprehension, and Use of Risk-Benefit Information. *Health Affairs.* 26(3):741–748.

Ropeik D, Gray G. 2002. *Risk: A Practical Guide for Deciding What's Really Safe and What's Really Dangerous in the World Around You.* New York: Houghton Mifflin.

Rothman RL, Housam R, Weiss H, Davis D, Gregory R, Gebretsadik T, et al. 2006. Patient Understanding of Food Labels: The Role of Literacy and Numeracy. *American Journal of Preventative Medicine.* 31(5):391–398.

Rothman RL, Montori VM, Cherrington A, Pignone MP. 2008. Perspective: The Role of Numeracy in Health Care. *Journal of Health Communication.* 13(6):583–595.

Schwartz LM, Woloshin S, Welch HG. 1999. Risk Communication in Clinical Practice: Putting Cancer in Context. *Journal of the National Cancer Institute. Monographs.* (25):124–133.

Wolff K, Cavanaugh K, Malone R, Hawk V, Gregory BP, Davis D, et al. 2009. The Diabetes Literacy and Numeracy Education Toolkit (DNET): Materials to Facilitate Diabetes Education and Management in Patients with Low Literacy and Numeracy Skills. *Diabetes Educator.* 35(2):233-236.

Woloshin S, Schwartz LM, Welch HG. 2002. Risk Charts: Putting Cancer in Context. *Journal of the National Cancer Institute.* 94(11):799-804.

Woloshin S, Schwartz LM, Welch HG. 2007. The Effectiveness of a Primer to Help People Understand Risk: Two Randomized Trials in Distinct Populations. *Annals of Internal Medicine.* 146(4):256-265.

Woloshin S, Schwartz LM, Welch HG. 2008. *Know Your Chances: Understanding Health Statistics.* Berkeley: University of California Press.

Organizational Efforts: Health Literacy at the Community, State, and National Levels

STARTING POINTS

Health literacy initiatives often begin with just one person (you, perhaps) who is a "health literacy advocate." An advocate needs no convincing why health literacy matters. This person's "job," nearly always as a volunteer, is to raise other people's awareness about health literacy and encourage needed action.

One person is often the way that health literacy initiatives begin. But it usually takes a team to make a sustainable, long-term difference. Many teams start internally with employees, staff, and customers from within an organization. A good mix of team members includes subject-matter experts (like clinicians, educators, and administrators), producers of health materials (such as writers and Web developers), and people representing the intended audience (including patients, families, and community members).

As teams experience success, they may branch out into the community with the goal of creating a broader, more unified approach for health literacy. For instance, a medical center might create an ongoing program of working with a local literacy program to test the readability of new patient education materials.

From there, community-based teams may unite as regional, statewide, multistate, and even national coalitions. Health Literacy Missouri is an example of a statewide organization that is not only leading the way locally but also helping to form regional partnerships and a national coalition. Arthur Culbert, PhD, is President of Health Literacy Missouri. He says that Health Literacy Missouri began thanks to a visionary physician who recognized the importance and scope of health literacy. From there, a committed board of directors allocated significant funding from its foundation. Health Literacy Missouri is now its own nonprofit organization that reaches out across state boundaries. As Culbert said in a *Health Literacy Out Loud* podcast, "It takes a village to make sweeping changes that not only save dollars, but also lives" (Osborne 2009, June 23).

And as I know from my many years leading Health Literacy Month, which occurs each October, there is no need for health literacy efforts to stop at geographic borders. Indeed, Health Literacy Month has been used worldwide to raise awareness since 1999.

STRATEGIES, IDEAS, AND SUGGESTIONS

Here are some ideas to consider (Osborne 2008; 2009, June 23; 2009, November 23):

Create a strategic vision. To me, health literacy is an opportunity to "dream big." Remember, the ultimate goal is a world in which patients and providers always understand one another. What will it take to help your organization become a part of this world? Do not worry if what you want feels too big or overwhelming. Just break it all down into "bite-sized" components. Then think about how to accomplish each component one by one.

Bring together people from varied professions, programs, and points of view. Here are some people you might want to include on your health literacy team:

- **"Worker bees."** This is a term I use when referring to those who actively help with day-to-day tasks. I am proud of the many years I spent as a "worker bee" as a psychiatric occupational therapist and chair of our hospital's patient and family education committee.
- **Department representatives.** Ideally, they will come from a wide range of departments, such as clinical services, marketing, risk management, information technology, and the library. They not only bring various perspectives but also can carry back the message that health literacy matters to their departments.
- **Patients and their families.** As you choose members, try to include those who represent your intended audience in terms of literacy,

age, disability, language, culture, and personal experience. They bring a unique perspective of those on the receiving end of health communication.

- **Representatives from community services.** Consider nearby organizations that also communicate health information. They might include the library, senior center, adult education program, and public safety departments.
- **Influential others.** Senior executives, well-respected community members, politicians, and local business owners not only add visibility to your efforts but also can act as champions to help sustain your efforts. Recruit them to be part of your team.

Partner with outside organizations. When looking for organizations to form partnerships with, think about groups you know that face communication challenges similar to yours or those that share a vision matching the one you have chosen to address. Here are some considerations when searching for potential partners:

- *Hospitals, health centers, and outpatient clinics* need to create and maintain effective patient education materials as well as develop programs that will enhance patient adherence to treatment regimens.
- *Public health initiatives* need to communicate messages that can be understood by a wide range of audiences.
- *Adult education or family literacy programs* focus their efforts on working with people to develop skills they need to function in their everyday life.
- *Immigrant services organizations* work to help people get beyond language and cultural barriers that can interfere with effective communication.
- *Cultural organizations* want people to be able to maintain the richness of their cultural heritage without being penalized because others don't understand them.
- *Advocacy groups* strive to have the needs of the people they represent not only heard, but also understood.
- *Health professional associations* are focused on finding ways to help their members become better providers.
- *Government departments and services* need to make and implement policies that provide for the well-being of their constituencies.

Make a compelling business case for health literacy. While it certainly is possible to accomplish tasks on a modest budget, most sustainable programs need a realistic investment of time and money. I've learned from many years of experience that we need to make a compelling case why health literacy matters, not just to advocates but also to funders.

The reality is that most health literacy initiatives compete for funding with other compelling programs. You can help by showing how health literacy impacts an organization's "bottom line." For instance, you might point out to a business that investing in health literacy can improve the wellness of its workforce. For hospitals and health centers, you might link health literacy concepts with the organization's mission, vision, and commitment to its community. (Read more in "Business Side of Health Literacy" starting on page 23.)

Stories from Practice: Healthcare Organizations and Literacy Programs Working Together

Dr. Winston Lawrence oversees a health literacy initiative sponsored by the Literacy Assistance Center (LAC) in New York City. In a *Health Literacy Out Loud* podcast, he talked about how this program brings together healthcare organizations and literacy professionals for the shared goal of improving the health of immigrants and adult learners throughout New York City.

This community collaboration offers learning for everyone: Literacy teachers help healthcare providers learn more about teaching, healthcare providers support teachers in educating about health, and adult literacy students gain practical experience in accessing and using health services while furthering their literacy and language skills.

For instance, as a result of this collaboration, students learned how to do tasks such as using a phone tree (press 1, 2) when calling for a medical appointment. They also learned how to read and correctly follow prescription labels. Lawrence is delighted how much this collaboration helps. As one student said, "I'm not afraid any more. Now I can talk with doctors."

Source: Osborne (2009, November 23).

 One person is often the way that health literacy initiatives begin. But it usually takes a team to make a sustainable, long-term difference.

CITATIONS

Osborne H. 2008. *Health Literacy Month Handbook: The Event Planning Guide for Health Literacy Advocates.* Available at http://healthliteracy.com/hlmonth-handbook. Accessed February 5, 2011.

Osborne H (host). 2009, June 23. Dr. Arthur Culbert Talks About Statewide Health Literacy Initiatives [audio podcast]. *Health Literacy Out Loud,* no. 17. Available at http://www.healthliteracy.com/hlol-statewide-initiatives. Accessed February 5, 2011.

Osborne H (host). 2009, November 23. Applying Adult Education Principles to Medicine and Public Health [audio podcast]. *Health Literacy Out Loud,* no. 28. Available at http://www.healthliteracy.com/hlol-adult-education. Accessed February 5, 2011.

SOURCES TO LEARN MORE

Health Literacy Month, www.healthliteracymonth.org.

Literacy Assistance Center. *Healthy Relationships: A Guide to Forming Partnerships Between Health Care Providers and Adult Education Programs.* Available at http://www.lacnyc.org/resources/healthlit/. Accessed February 6, 2011.

Lloyd LLJ, Ammary NJ, Epstein LG, Johnson R, Rhee K. 2006. A Transdisciplinary Approach to Improve Health Literacy and Reduce Disparities. *Health Promotion Practice.* (3):331–335.

Osborne H. 2008, July 24. In Other Words . . . Bridging Literacy and Language Differences for Better Health Outcomes. *On Call.* Available at http://www.healthliteracy.com/literacy-language-differences. Accessed February 6, 2011.

Osborne H (host). 2010, January 5. Making a Business Case to Move Health Literacy Forward [audio podcast]. *Health Literacy Out Loud,* no. 30. Available at http://www.healthliteracy.com/hlol-business-case. Accessed February 5, 2011.

Osborne H. 2011. *Checklists for Health Literacy Month Events.* Available at http://healthliteracy.com/hlmonth-checklists. Accessed July 10, 2011.

Plain Language

Plain language (or "plain English") helps everyone—not just readers who have limited literacy or limited English skills. According to Plain Language Association International (2011), "Plain language is communication designed to meet the needs of the intended audience, so people can understand information that is important to their lives."

Writing in plain language is both a science and an art. The "science" part has to do with following established guidelines and using proven strategies. The "art" has to do with putting information together in ways that are not only understandable but also inviting, appealing, useful, and relevant. Writing in plain language probably isn't the hardest job you've ever done. But don't be surprised—it may not be the easiest either. I've learned from many years of experience that it is often hard to be simple.

Sometimes writers worry that plain-language wording will insult stronger readers. Or that content is so simplified that it dilutes a more nuanced message. While appreciating these concerns, I do not share them. To me, plain language is not "dumbing down" but rather smartening up, providing information in ways that most everyone can understand. Below is an example.

Stories from Practice: Before and After Examples

Here is a "before" and "after" example of flu vaccine information from 2009 (when two flu shots were needed, not just one). Which version do you find easier to read, understand, and act on?

"Before" example of original text:

What You Should Know and Do This Flu Season If You Are 65 Years and Older. The best way to prevent the flu is with a flu vaccine. People 65 years and older are recommended for annual seasonal flu vaccination. People 65 and older who have not yet gotten a seasonal flu vaccine should still seek vaccination, although supplies of seasonal flu vaccine are limited because of early availability of, and high interest in, seasonal flu vaccine this year. People 65 years and older are now encouraged to seek vaccination against 2009 H1N1 vaccine. Supplies of the vaccines to protect against the 2009 H1N1 virus have increased dramatically and most places have opened up vaccination to anyone who wants it. This vaccine is the best way to protect against the 2009 H1N1 pandemic virus. Those who have been patiently waiting to receive the 2009 H1N1 vaccine, including people 65 years and older, are now encouraged to get vaccinated.

"After" example in plain language:

Know what to do about the flu. The best way you can help prevent the flu is by getting two flu shots. One is a shot to prevent the seasonal (winter) flu. The other is a shot to prevent a new flu called H1N1.

The U.S. Centers for Disease Control (CDC) recommends that people who are at least 65 years old get both shots. You may have heard a while ago that there was not enough flu vaccine. That has changed and there now is enough vaccine for everyone who wants flu shots. There is no need to wait. Get your flu shots today.

Source: "Before" example from Centers for Disease Control and Prevention (2010). Available at http://www.cdc.gov/h1n1flu/65andolder .htm. "After" example written in plain language by Helen Osborne.

STRATEGIES, IDEAS, AND SUGGESTIONS

Here are some plain language strategies you could use (Osborne 2009, August 3; 2009, December 7; 2010, March 13):

Build a team. It takes a team to write a readable document. To me, this team should include: a plain-language writer who is skilled in plain language and an unceasing advocate for readers; one or more content experts who determine information that must stay or can go; and readers who represent your intended audience in terms of literacy level, language, age, culture, and interest in and familiarity with the subject matter.

Identify project goals. Whether you are working on your own project or writing for someone else, identify goals from the start. I do this by asking what readers should know, do, and feel as a result of reading this document. I jot down the answers, refer to them while writing, and review these goals at the project's end.

Organize content in ways that make sense to your readers:

- *Identify one primary message and support it with a limited number of (usually three to five) key points.* Obviously, when you write in plain language you can't include everything because documents would be too long. Instead, prioritize "need-to-know" skills and behaviors that readers must learn rather than "nice-to-know" background information that is less essential.
- *Organize key points in ways that make sense to readers (not just writers).* Generally, this means starting with the concept of "what's in it for me" (WIIFM), which is a brief statement about why people should read this information. When writing about a new surgical procedure, for example, begin with how patients can benefit from this procedure rather than how many awards your medical facility has received. At the end, summarize key points and include non-print resources (phone numbers, places to go) as well as written and Web-based materials.
- *Have ways for readers to interact with written materials.* Options include check-off boxes, fill-in-the-blank exercises, and short quizzes. You can also have lines or spaces for patients to write their provider's name or appointment time.

Use understandable words:

- *Use common one- or two-syllable words.* It can be hard to choose the "just right" words, especially when writing medical information with lots of technical, multisyllabic terms. If possible, use common one- and two-syllable words that people know and already understand. An example is "heart attack" instead of "myocardial infarction."

- *Define unfamiliar, yet necessary, words and terms.* Certainly there are times when you need a more technical term. If so, define it, show the correct pronunciation, and include a simply worded example or explanation. For instance, "Bronchitis, bron-ki-tis, a disease that makes you cough."

- *Be consistent, using the exact same wording each time.* Choose one term and use it consistently. For example, if you choose "bandage," then use it throughout the booklet rather than adding "Band-Aids," "gauze," and "compresses."

- *Be cautious when using contractions like "don't" and "you'll."* Though contractions like these sound friendly and conversational, people with limited reading skills or those learning English may not understand them. Instead, write out the full words, as in "do not" and "you will."

- *Be sensitive to concepts, category, and value judgment words.* Though familiar, these types of words can be difficult as readers may not have a framework to understand their meaning (Doak, Doak, & Root 1996)
  - Concept words. These describe general or abstract ideas like "wellness" and "health status."
  - Category words. These include overall groupings, such as "poultry," rather than specifying chicken or turkey. Or "health professionals" or "healthcare providers" instead of specifying disciplines and job titles.
  - Value judgment words. These refer to amounts or thresholds that readers must determine, such as "rarely" and "moderate."

Write succinct sentences:

- *Vary sentence length and style.* Yes, it is possible to be clear and simple but not boring. Mix up your sentence length and style just a bit. For instance, instead of always writing choppy sentences like "Take 4 pills before breakfast. Eat breakfast. Go for a 30-minute walk," you could write, "Start your day in a healthy way. Take 4 pills before you eat breakfast. Then go for a 30-minute walk after you finish eating."

- *Have just one main idea and no more than about 15 words in each sentence.* This lessens the chance of having complex sentences with lots of commas and clauses. Instead of overly long sentences, you might use bullet points (such as I've done throughout this book).

- *Identify who is doing the action.* Use an active sentence structure to make clear who does what. An example is "Pat is baking a cream pie." The passive and harder-to-read version is "A cream pie is being baked by Pat."
- *Be sensitive to conditional if/then sentences.* Health care is filled with lots of "iffy" conditional information, with sentences starting with "if" and having "then" in the middle. But such sentences can be hard to understand as readers must comprehend the "if" clause, the "then" clause, and the relationship between the two. When writing a lot of conditional information, consider using a simple table. Here is an example from an Easy Read article I "translated" into plain language for the Amputee Coalition.

When You Take a Shower or Bath

Problem	What you can do
If you have trouble stepping into or out of the bathtub or shower . . .	Then . . .
If you cannot stand when you take a shower or bath . . .	Then . . .
If you have trouble transferring into and out of the tub . . .	Then . . .
If you cannot carry your bath supplies (such as shampoo and soap) . . .	Then . . .
If you are afraid you might fall when getting into or out of the shower or bath . . .	Then . . .
If you cannot feel heat, cold, or pain . . .	Then . . .
If you cannot easily move in the shower or bath . . .	Then . . .

Source: Osborne (2008, September/October).

Use an engaging tone:

- *Write in a friendly and conversational tone, though not overly chatty or cute.* Tone should match the content—sad or difficult subjects should not be treated lightly.
- *Write as though you were talking, using personal pronouns like "you" and "your."* One way to achieve this is by reading aloud as you write and edit.
- *Present information in as positive a manner as possible.* For example, start with what patients can do, rather than what they can not. But also be honest. Don't refer to a medicine as a "pleasantly flavored drink" when it really tastes like chalk.
- *Be clear and specific, not asking readers to guess or assume what to do.* For example, write "take two ten-minute walks each day" rather than "exercise moderately."

Consider format and layout:

- *Write in a font size that is large enough to see.* Generally, this is 12-point type; 14- or 16-point type is preferable when writing for older readers or those who have limited vision. Avoid stylized or italic letters and instead use more traditional type such as Times New Roman or Arial.
- *Use a combination of upper and lower case, rather than all capital letters.* This way, readers get visual cues about the letters they see.
- *Justify (line up) words on the left, not centered or on the right.* Centered text often results in uneven spacing that makes reading difficult. Also, when lines all begin at the same place on the left, readers know where to focus first.
- *Allow adequate white space.* Generally this is about a 50/50 split between printed and non-printed areas. Have margins that are at least an inch wide. This not only is easy on the eyes but also allows room for people to add notes, comments, questions, and doodles.
- *Have visual contrast between letters and background.* This usually is black type on white or light, non-glossy paper. When you make copies, make sure that the print is clean and easy to see. Sometimes, copies of copies are unreadable.
- *Use headers to identify main topics.* Often, the most informative ones are written as questions such as "What Is Diabetes?" (To learn more about format and layout, go to "Document Design," starting on page 51.)

Use graphics wisely:

- *Select graphics that are informative and not just decorative.* Sometimes, however, decorative designs are so appealing that they motivate people to read. When this is the case, use designs so long as they do not distract from the message.
- *Use recognizable images rather than abstract symbols that might be misunderstood.* For example, a red circle with a slash across it is commonly understood by people in the United States to mean "don't," but it may not be as familiar to those from other parts of the world.
- *Show and tell readers the correct way to perform tasks by having pictures with simple written captions beneath them.* This can be very effective, as when showing each step in a sequence of instructions.
- *Select pictures that are culturally relevant and appropriate to your audience.* An example is drawings of healthy, active seniors in a brochure for older adults.

- *Draw internal body parts in context of the entire body.* This not only conveys size and proportion, but also avoids "disembodied body parts," which people may find confusing or upsetting. To show detail, include an enlargement of the body part alongside the larger illustration. (Read more in "Visuals," starting on page 215.)

Confirm comprehension. The best way to determine whether readers can understand is by asking for feedback. Ask your intended readers to review drafts of your written material. Find out what they think about the document's organization, words, tone, layout, and graphics. Also ask how readers plan to use the information they just read. Allow sufficient time not only to make their recommended changes but also to test again to make sure you didn't introduce new problems. (Read more in "Confirming Understanding: Feedback," starting on page 35.)

 Writing in plain language probably isn't the hardest job you've ever done. But don't be surprised—it may not be the easiest either. I've learned from many years of experience that it is often hard to be simple.

CITATIONS

Centers for Disease Control and Prevention. 2010. Available at http://www.cdc.gov/h1n1flu/65andolder.htm. Accessed July 18, 2011.

Doak CC, Doak LG, Root JH. 1996. *Teaching Patients with Low Literacy Skills.* 2nd ed. Philadelphia: J. B. Lippincott. Available online at http://www.hsph.harvard.edu/healthliteracy/resources/doak-book/index.html. Accessed December 30, 2010.

Osborne H. 2008, September/October. Ways to Do Grooming and Bathing Tasks Alone. *inMotion Easy Read.* 15(5). Available at http://www.amputee-coalition.org/easyread/inmotion/sep_oct_05/grooming-ez.html.

Osborne H (host). 2009, August 3. Communicating Clearly on the Web [audio podcast]. *Health Literacy Out Loud,* no. 19. Available at http://healthliteracy.com/hlol-web. Accessed February 6, 2011.

Osborne H (host). 2009, December 7. Using Design to Get Readers to Read and Keep Reading [audio podcast]. *Health Literacy Out Loud,* no. 29. Available at http://healthliteracy.com/hlol-design-principles. Accessed February 6, 2011.

Osborne H (host). 2010, March 3. Creating Usable, Useful Health Websites for Readers at All Levels [audio podcast]. *Health Literacy Out Loud,* no. 34. Available at http://healthliteracy.com/hlol-websites-for-all-readers. Accessed February 6, 2011.

Plain Language Association International (PLAIN). 2011. Available at http://www.plainlanguagenetwork.org. Accessed February 6, 2011.

Sources to Learn More

Center for Plain Language, www.centerforplainlanguage.org.

Centers for Disease Control and Prevention. 2009. *Plain Language Thesaurus for Health Communications.* Available at http://www.plainlanguage.gov/populartopics/ health_literacy/index.cfm. Accessed February 6, 2011. (Fifth item under "Federal Agency Links about Health Literacy.")

Centers for Medicare and Medicaid Services, U.S. Department of Health and Human Services. 2010. *Toolkit for Making Written Material Clear and Effective.* Available at http://www.cms.gov/WrittenMaterialsToolkit/. Accessed January 8, 2011.

Cutts M. 2008. *Plain English Lexicon: A Guide to Whether Your Words Will Be Understood.* Plain Language Commission. Available at www.clearest.co.uk/?id=46. Accessed February 6, 2011.

Davis TC, Mayeaux EJ, Fredrickson D, Bocchini JA Jr, Jackson RH, Murphy PW. 1994. Reading Ability of Parents Compared with Reading Level of Pediatric Patient Education Materials. *Pediatrics.* 93(3):460–468.

Goldfarb NM, DuBay WH. 2006. Writing Good at a Seventh-Grade Reading Level. *Journal of Clinical Research Best Practices.* 2(1):1–4.

Kripalani S, Robertson R, Love-Ghaffari MH, Henderson LE, Praska J, Strawder A, et al. 2007. Development of an Illustrated Medication Schedule as a Low-Literacy Patient Education Tool. *Patient Education and Counseling.* 66(3): 368–377.

Maximus. 2005. *The Health Literacy Style Manual.* Available at http://www .coveringkidsandfamilies.org/resources/docs/stylemanual.pdf. Accessed April 21, 2011.

Osborne H. 2005, July. In Other Words . . . What Makes Web Sites "Patient Friendly?" *On Call.* Available at http://healthliteracy.com/patient-friendly-websites. Accessed February 6, 2011.

Osborne H. 2010. Writing in Plain Language: A Quick Guide from Start to Finish. *American Medical Writers Association Journal.* 25(4):169–171.

Plain Language Medical Dictionary (a project of the University of Michigan Taubman Health Sciences Library as part of the Michigan Health Literacy Awareness project). Available at http://www.lib.umich.edu/plain-language-dictionary.

Plain Writing Act of 2010, H.R. 946, 111th Cong. (2010). Available at http://www .govtrack.us/congress/bill.xpd?bill=h111-946. Accessed February 6, 2011.

Redish J. 2007. *Letting Go of the Words: Writing Web Content That Works.* Boston: Morgan Kaufmann.

Ridpath JR, Greene SM, Wiese CJ. 2007. *PRISM Readability Toolkit.* 3rd ed. Seattle: Group Health Research Institute. Available at http://www .grouphealthresearch.org/capabilities/readability/ghchs_readability_toolkit .pdf. Accessed February 6, 2011.

Roskos SK, Keenum AJ, Newman LM, Wallace LS. 2007. Literacy Demands and Formatting Characteristics of Opioid Contracts in Chronic Nonmalignant Pain Management. *Journal of Pain.* 8(10):753–758.

Stableford S, Mettger W. 2007. Plain Language: A Strategic Response to the Health Literacy Challenge. *Journal of Public Health Policy.* 28:71–93.

Sudore RL, Landefeld CS, Barnes DE, Lindquist K, Williams BA, Brody R, et al. 2007. An Advance Directive Redesigned to Meet the Literacy Level of Most Adults: A Randomized Trial. *Patient Education and Counseling.* 69(1–3), 165–195.

U.S. Department of Health and Human Services, Office of Disease Prevention and Health Promotion. 2011. *Health Communication Activities: Quick Guide to Health Literacy.* Available at http://www.health.gov/communication/literacy/quickguide/. Accessed February 6, 2011.

Wallace LS, Keenum AJ, Roskos SE, McDaniel KS. 2007. Development and Validation of a Low-Literacy Opioid Contract. *Journal of Pain.* 8(10):759–766.

Question-Asking

"Do you have any questions?" the provider asks. The patient shakes his head, indicating "no." While the provider might assume this response means she did a good job communicating, the patient may think this is a polite way of not saying how confused he really is.

Why is it so hard for patients to ask questions? It is hard for almost all patients, no matter how well educated, to think of questions to ask when sitting in an examining room, wearing only a skimpy hospital gown. "Asking questions is one of the most difficult tasks patients face," says Lisa Bernstein, who is Executive Director of the What to Expect Foundation, based in New York City. Bernstein often teaches providers how to help patients ask questions. She explains that asking questions is a learned skill, not an innate ability. For patients to ask, Bernstein says, they must be fluent in medical vocabulary, understand basic biology, and have enough confidence to speak up to respected health professionals (Osborne 2006).

Question-asking can also be influenced by emotions and culture. It might be that patients do not ask questions because they feel scared and overwhelmed, or fear asking a "stupid" question. This reluctance may also be cultural or generational, as when people believe (like my mother did) that it is rude to question those in authority.

Why is question-asking so important? Health literacy and patient safety experts agree that question-asking brings many benefits, including helping people learn new content, confirming they understand key concepts, and framing information within a more personal context.

What are some strategies to help patients ask questions? There are several initiatives to help patients ask questions. These include AskMe3 from the Partnership for Clear Health Communications at the National Patient Safety Foundation and Questions Are the Answer from AHRQ (Agency for Healthcare Research and Quality). AskMe3 has three simple questions that patients are encouraged to ask, and that providers should answer, in every health care interaction. The questions are:

- "What is my main problem?"
- "What do I need to do about it?"
- "Why is it important for me to do this?" (National Patient Safety Foundation)

In presentations to consumers, I find that participants are very receptive to these three questions and refer to them often. But are these three questions effective? In an early study with patients who already ask a lot of questions and have high levels of adherence, data showed "no evidence that the AM3 intervention results in patients asking their physicians a greater number of questions or more specific questions" (Galliher, et al. 2010).

Carolyn M. Clancy, MD, is director of AHRQ. She says that her agency created Questions Are the Answer to help reduce the number of preventable harms happening to patients each year. Questions Are the Answer builds on a concept that patients and providers agree is important—that patients should be involved in their own health care. Dr. Clancy says that involved patients tend to have better health outcomes, and asking questions is an important, though admittedly basic, way to be involved. "Yes, it is straightforward. But people don't do it," says Clancy (Osborne 2008, June 25).

Given that a patient's time with the doctor is often short, Clancy adds that it is important for patients to make priorities in their list of questions and find out how to ask additional questions after the visit ends (Clancy 2010).

A resource to help is the Questions Are the Answer Web site (http://www.ahrq.gov/questionsaretheanswer/; available in Spanish at http://www.ahrq.gov/superheroes/getinfo.htm). It includes

- "Helpful Tips" consumers can use when communicating with their providers, along with links to learn more.

- Videos and public service announcements with a humorous yet compelling message about the importance of asking questions.
- "Build Your Question List" with core information that providers need to communicate and patients must understand. Consumers can select which questions to ask and then print their list. This printout even includes space to write the answers.

STRATEGIES, IDEAS, AND SUGGESTIONS

Here are some strategies you might put into practice (Osborne 2006; 2008, June 25; 2008, November 3):

Invite, or even insist, on questions. According to Donald Rubin, PhD, who is an expert on oral communication, one of the most useful things that providers can say is, "*Please* ask me a question or two that you have been wondering about. You don't bother me when you ask questions. In fact, you help me do my job better when you ask questions. I really like it when my patients can come up with a question or two to ask me." Rubin says that this "almost insistent invitation to ask questions is important because so many people want to be 'good patients,' and believe that being a good patient means not bothering the doctor" (Rubin 2010).

Rubin adds one more bit of advice for providers, "Get to the point of an answer without too much elaboration. And then check to make sure you answered the question that the patient really wanted answered." Rubin suggests doing so with your own questions such as, "Does that get at what you were asking?" Or "Is there any follow-up information you feel you need now?" (Rubin 2011).

Elicit questions with open-ended phrasing. Ask questions in ways that encourage a range of responses, such as "What are your questions?" This open-ended phrasing lets patients know that questions are expected, as opposed to the close-ended (yes/no) phrasing "Do you have any questions?"

Offer reassurance. Help patients feel more at ease by letting them know that they can ask any question they want. When patients sheepishly admit they have some "stupid questions," reassure them that there are no "bad" (rather than "stupid") questions. Indeed, you've most likely heard all these questions before.

Ask as well as answer. When patients have no questions, ask some of your own. For instance, when a patient comes in for an angioplasty, you might ask, "Why you are here today?" If the patient answers with something quite basic, such as "because of a bad leg," then follow up with more specific questions. These may focus on recent symptoms or the patient's understanding of the procedure. This question-and-answer format invariably leads to a fuller discussion.

Prepare commonly asked questions. Lisa Bernstein of the What to Expect Foundation works with providers at prenatal clinics who often see women with limited education or literacy and language skills. Frequently, these women are reluctant to ask questions. One strategy that Bernstein recommends is for providers to prepare questions that women commonly ask in routine prenatal visits. Then, when a woman says she has no questions,

---

Stories from Practice: Encouraging Others to Ask Questions

Ms. Winona Love volunteers as a "Health Literacy Coach" for the Meals On Wheels program run by the Senior Center in Blakely, Georgia. She not only delivers meals to homebound elders but also encourages "customers" to ask questions when going to their doctors. From her own experience as well as from experience helping others, Ms. Love feels strongly that question-asking helps people understand what is wrong and how to take care of health problems.

But sometimes people don't ask questions. Ms. Love thinks this can happen because people don't jot down their questions ahead of time and then cannot remember what they wanted to ask. Also, some people are embarrassed to ask questions that doctors might think are dumb. And many people want to respect the doctor's busy schedule and not take up too much time asking questions.

Here is some advice that Ms. Love shares with her customers:

- Ask what is wrong with you. Find out why you are having this problem. And if the doctor gives you new medicine, ask what it's for.
- When you think about what to ask, write your questions down. Then, when you get in the doctor's office, you'll know what to say.
- It doesn't matter how dumb you think your question is. It's not. Ask your doctor about it. When it comes to health, no question is dumb.

Source: Love (2010).

the provider can readily say, "A lot of women in their (x) month of pregnancy ask about . . . . Is that a question you want me to answer?" Bernstein finds that doing so starts a dialogue about important health information and also models good question-asking behavior (Osborne 2006, November/December).

Encourage patients to write down their questions. Make it easier for patients by providing pens and paper in waiting areas as well as examining rooms. As needed, add a clipboard or other hard writing surface—I know from experience it's mighty hard to write when the only available surface is a squishy exam table.

Consider the expense of not asking questions. Do you fear that answering a patient's questions will take too long? If so, consider the added time and expense when patients call the office to clarify information, do not follow directions, or have a preventable problem that might have been avoided if only patients knew what to do.

 Health literacy and patient safety experts agree that question-asking brings many benefits, including helping people learn new content, confirming they understand key concepts, and framing information within a more personal context.

CITATIONS

Clancy C. 2010. Personal communication.

Galliher JM, Post DM, Weiss BD, Dickinson LM, Manning BK, Staton EW, et al. 2010. Patients' Question-Asking Behavior During Primary Care Visits: A Report from the AAFP National Research Network. *Annals of Family Medicine* 8(2):151–159.

Love W. 2010. Telephone interview.

National Patient Safety Foundation. 2011. *AskMe3*. Available at http://www.npsf .org/askme3/. Accessed July 10, 2011.

Osborne H. 2006, November/December. In Other Words . . . Helping Patients Ask Questions. *On Call*. Available at http://www.healthliteracy.com/asking-questions. Accessed February 6, 2011.

Osborne H. 2008, June 25. In Other Words . . . "Questions Are the Answer" to Helping Patients Understand Their Health. *On Call*. Available at http://www .healthliteracy.com/question-asking. Accessed February 6, 2011.

Osborne H (host). 2008, November 3. Lisa Bernstein Talks About Patient-Centered Communication. *Health Literacy Out Loud,* no. 4. Available at http://healthliteracy.com/hlol-patient-centered-communication. Accessed February 6, 2011.

Rubin D. 2010. Personal communication.
Rubin D. 2011. Personal communication.

SOURCES TO LEARN MORE

Center for Health and Risk Communication. 2011. *Health Literacy on Wheels.* Athens, GA: University of Georgia. Available at http://chrc.uga.edu/research/. Accessed February 6, 2011.

Katz MG, Jacobson TA, Veledar E, Kripalani S. 2007. Patient Literacy and Question-Asking Behavior During the Medical Encounter: A Mixed-Methods Analysis. *Journal of General Internal Medicine.* 22:782–786.

Kinnersley P, Edwards A, Hood K, Ryan R, Prout H, Cadbury N, et al. 2008. Interventions Before Consultations to Help Patients Address Their Information Needs by Encouraging Question Asking: Systematic Review. *British Medical Journal.* 337:a485. Available at http://www.bmj.com/cgi/content/full/337/jul16_1/a485. Accessed July 10, 2010.

Regulatory and Legal Language

STARTING POINTS

Regulatory and medical-legal documents, such as research informed consent documents, HIPAA (Health Insurance Portability and Accountability Act) materials, and institutional administrative or procedural forms, are notoriously difficult to read and understand. Many are written at college reading levels or beyond and filled with "legalese" and medical jargon—a combination understood mostly by lawyers, administrators, and bureaucrats.

Mark Hochhauser, PhD, is a nationally known readability expert who knows a lot about informed consent documents. He says that beyond difficult words and concepts, many informed consent documents have so much information that readers can easily get overwhelmed. For example, the U.S. Food and Drug Administration (FDA) requires that informed consent documents for research have eight basic elements (topics or subjects) plus six "when needed" ones.

Hochhauser says that some of these elements are quite technical, such as descriptions of research drugs and their potential side effects. When informed consent forms are for research and must include items required for HIPAA, Hochhauser says there can be 14 to 26 separate elements—a hefty amount of information for readers at all levels (Hochhauser 2011).

Strategies, Ideas, and Suggestions

Here are some ideas to consider (Hochhauser 2011; Osborne 2005; 2009):

Organize information from easiest to more complex. While the content of medical-legal documents may be mandated by in-house policies or outside agencies, the order in which information is presented is generally not. To improve readability:

- Consider starting as newspapers do with basic information about who, what, when, where, why, and how.
- Include an introductory statement about why this information is relevant to readers. Some refer to this as WIIFM, "What's In It For Me."
- Present easiest information first, followed by more complex. You can do this for the entire document as well as within each section.
- Provide a "layered notice." This is a brief (one- or two-page) summary of key points written in plain language. You can attach this summary to the more complex legal document.

Apply the principles of plain language. Whenever possible:

- Write in a conversational style using terms like "you" (the patient) and "we" (the organization or provider).
- Explain new concepts by putting them into context and giving examples. These concepts include important terms such as "risk" and "benefits." I frequently describe risk as "problems that sometimes happen" and benefits as "ways that this (medication, treatment, or procedure) can help."
- Design documents so that readers can easily find the information they need. One way is by having headers clearly indicating each section.
- Use common words that people already know. This means using words like "choice" instead of "alternative" and "tell us" rather than "notify." To make this task easier, consider creating an in-house glossary of acceptable substitute words.
- Define only those words that need defining. If you are uncertain about which words to define, test them with intended readers or at least get an opinion from outsiders.
- Show words with close variations in parentheses. An example is " 'Co-payment' (sometimes called 'co-insurance' or 'co-pay')."

Read more in "Plain Language," starting on page 157.

Stories from Practice: Complex Legal Language

I often lead plain-language workshops for health professionals. While participants are almost always enthused and eager to use their new plain-language writing skills, invariably someone will ask how to respond when administrators and lawyers insist on complex legal language.

To learn about this, I spoke with Joseph Kimble, a law professor at Thomas Cooley Law School in Lansing, Michigan. He is a champion of plain language and author of numerous articles and the book *Lifting the Fog of Legalese*.

According to Kimble, it is a myth that traditional legal language is needed to protect an organization if a case is brought against it. He says that if a plain-language version of information has the same content and substantive meaning, then an organization will get exactly the same protection.

Kimble also says that documents do not need stuffy words such as "thereof" and "pursuant to." While acknowledging the need for certain legal content, Kimble firmly believes that most information can be explained in ways ordinary citizens can understand. If your organization's lawyer insists on certain wording, you (the plain language writer) should ask why. Find out if particular wording is required by statute or regulation. Ask for its citation number in the *Code of Federal Regulations* (or whatever other source the lawyer is referencing) and then look up the requirements. You can often do this without assistance from a lawyer, says attorney Joseph Kimble.

Source: Osborne (2009, January 29).

Encourage readers to take action. Provide spaces below key content with directions to "write any questions you have about what you just read." Also, ask readers to circle any words they do not know the meaning of or do not fully understand. This way, you can be more aware of words and concepts to discuss with patients in greater detail.

Remember that patients may be reading an informed consent document for the first and only time. The purpose of informed consent is twofold: (1) to inform the patient(s) about a medical procedure so they can make an informed decision, and (2) to obtain legal consent for the provider to perform it. When providers do the same procedure hundreds or thousands of times, it can be easy to forget that patients might be reading this document only once.

Create an environment in which people can ask for help. Make sure that the environment in which people are asked to read and sign legal forms feels private and is secure. For example, if you ask patients to write phone numbers on a form, then have a way to shred copies they discard because of errors. Be sensitive to people's emotional states, as well. For sure, it is difficult for patients to concentrate on complex information when they are sick, anxious, or pre-medicated for a procedure. One way to help is by offering to read documents aloud.

Many regulatory and legal documents are written at college reading levels or beyond and filled with "legalese" and medical jargon—a combination understood mostly by lawyers, administrators, and bureaucrats.

CITATIONS

Hochhauser M. 2011. Personal communication.

Osborne H. 2005, September. In Other Words . . . Clearing a Path . . . Helping Patients Understand Medical-Legal Information. *On Call.* http://www.healthliteracy.com/medical-legal. Accessed February 8, 2011.

Osborne H. 2009, January 29. In Other Words: Working with Lawyers to Make Health Information Clear. *On Call.* Available at http://www.healthliteracy.com/legal-information. Accessed February 8, 2011.

SOURCES TO LEARN MORE

AHRQ (Agency for Healthcare Research and Quality). 2009. *The AHRQ Informed Consent and Authorization Toolkit for Minimal Risk Research.* AHRQ Publication No. 09-0089-EF. Available at http://www.ahrq.gov/fund/informedconsent/. Accessed July 7, 2010.

Brandes WL, Furnas S, McClellan F. 1996. *Literacy, Health, and the Law: An Exploration of the Law and the Plight of Marginal Reader Within the Healthcare System.* Philadelphia: Health Promotion Council of Southeastern Pennsylvania.

Code of Federal Regulations. Available at http://www.gpoaccess.gov/cfr/index.html.

Goldfarb NM, DuBay W. 2006. Informed Consent Form Makeover. *Journal of Clinical Research Best Practices.* 2(5): 1–3. Available at http://firstclinical.com/journal/2006/0605_Makeover.pdf. Accessed February 8, 2011.

Health Resources and Services Administration of the U.S. Department of Health and Human Services. 2009. *Plain Language Principles and Thesaurus for Making HIPAA Privacy Notices More Readable.* Washington, DC: Government Printing Office. Available at http://www.aspiruslibrary.org/literacy/ MakingHIPAAPrivacyNoticesMoreReadable.pdf. Accessed June 29, 2011.

Hochhauser M. 2008. Designing More Legible Consent Forms. *SoCRA Source: A Publication of the Society of Clinical Research Associates.* 57:62–63.

Hochhauser M. 2008. Too Many Unnecessary Words = Confusing Consent Forms. *SoCRA Source: A Publication of the Society of Clinical Research Associates.* 56:58–59.

Kimble J. 1994–95. Answering the Critics of Plain Language. *Scribes Journal of Legal Writing.* 5:51–85. Available at http://www.plainlanguagenetwork.org/kimble/ critics.htm. Accessed February 8, 2011.

Kimble J. 2006. *Lifting the Fog of Legalese: Essays on Plain Language.* Durham, NC: Carolina Academic Press.

Landro L. 2008, February 6. The Informed Patient: Consent Forms That Patients Can Understand. *Wall Street Journal Online.* Available at http://online.wsj.com/ article/SB120224055435844931.html. Accessed February 8, 2011.

Paasche-Orlow MK, Jacob DM, Hochhauser M, Parker RM. 2009. National Survey of Patients' Bill of Rights Statutes. *Journal of General Internal Medicine.* 24(4):489–494.

Stories

STARTING POINTS

Stories are powerful health communication tools. Combining emotions and facts, stories help people connect with health information in a very personal way. Audiences of all ages and cultures relate to stories because they help people bridge differences and find qualities they have in common. Stories are not only engaging and entertaining, but also easy for most everyone to understand—even those who have trouble reading or paying attention.

Distinct from other types of communication, stories have a beginning, middle, and end, though not always in that order. They also have characters (real or imagined) who convey feelings and communicate ideas. While stories should always contain essential truths (the points you are trying to convey), all the details do not need to be factual (such as changing a character's name or setting where the story took place).

You can tell a story to one person or to many, to professionals or the lay public, to children or adults, in formal as well as more relaxed settings. For most people, albeit not everyone, a well-told story is almost always welcome. Here's my story about understanding the power of stories: I met Senator Edward M. "Ted" Kennedy many years ago at an event about healthcare reform. We spoke briefly and I asked about his commitment to health care. Senator Kennedy responded by telling me stories about his family's health care—including his mother's home health care, his son's leg amputation, and his own experience with a broken back. Beyond hearing why health care issues mattered so much to him, I also learned that even a U.S. senator knows the power of personal stories.

STRATEGIES, IDEAS, AND SUGGESTIONS

Here are some ways to use stories in practice (Osborne 2002; 2008):

Tell stories. When telling stories in healthcare settings, make sure the stories are relevant and true, do not violate anyone's privacy, and are not told simply to be entertaining. Sometimes, you will need to make clear why you are telling the story, perhaps by saying, "Let me tell you about someone with a health history like yours who . . ." Other times, the reason for the story is evident. Stories don't always have to be spoken. Indeed, like in this book, stories are sprinkled throughout to clarify key points and make them "come alive."

Encourage patients to share stories. By listening to stories, providers can learn a lot about their patients' strengths, concerns, and points of view. You can encourage patients to tell you stories by saying "Tell me about a time that . . ." or "Give me an example of the problems you have when . . . "

Help patients focus on the point of a story. Telling stories needn't take a long time. If you feel that patients are talking in too roundabout a way, help them focus by saying something like, "You started talking about your heart and now you're telling me about your feet. Please tell me more about how these problems connect." Being directive like this is preferable to asking patients to be "brief," which may cause them to filter out details that may or may not be important.

Listen for what's missing in a story. When listening to stories—especially ones told by patients—consider the story in its entirety. If the story doesn't make sense, find out what is missing or what is wrong. Encourage patients to listen to their own stories, as well. It's likely that the version they tell you differs in some way from the one they share with family and friends. Make sure you understand patients' stories correctly, perhaps by saying, "Let me tell you what I've heard," or "Correct me if I have any of the details wrong." And, of course, thank patients for sharing their stories.

Decide whether to share stories from your own experience. Whether you use stories in clinical practice or in educational settings, there are risks and benefits in talking about your own experiences. When you share your story, you run the risk of taking attention away from the points you are trying to make or the person you are caring for. But, used carefully and told well, stories can be very effective ways for patients and health providers to get their points across and better understand what the other has to say.

Stories from Practice: Healthcare Stories Used in Many Ways

Kevin Brooks, PhD, is co-author of *Storytelling for User Experience* (Quesenbery & Brooks 2010). He also is a storyteller and storytelling coach. Brooks and I spoke about stories in health care, and he highlighted four ways they are often used:

- *Health providers tell stories to patients.* Providers may use stories to raise awareness about general health or wellness issues, or to focus more specifically on an illness and its treatment. An example is a story about how Helen works at a computer all day but has fewer neck aches now that she regularly goes to a fitness center.
- *Patients tell stories to health providers.* Perhaps prompted by their providers, patients can tell stories about what it's like to live with a particular disease or condition. Providers should listen carefully to what patients do and do not say. By listening, providers are likely to hear about the patient's physical, psychological, and emotional state, all woven together.
- *Health professionals tell stories to health professionals.* Whether called case studies, vignettes, or scenarios, stories include not only facts and figures but also values. This can be of great benefit, especially when talking to colleagues of different disciplines or points of view.
- *Patients tell stories to patients.* When people hear a story being told, they connect with the teller in a personal way—getting the sense that the teller is "just like me." This happens regardless of whether the storyteller is famous (perhaps an actor or political figure) or anonymous (like a member of a self-help group).

Source: Brooks (2004).

 You can tell a story to one person or to many, to professionals or the lay public, to children or adults, in formal as well as more relaxed settings. For most people, albeit not everyone, a well-told story is almost always welcome.

CITATIONS

Brooks K. 2004. Personal communication.

Osborne H. 2002. In Other Words . . . Narrative Power . . . Using Stories in Healthcare Communication, *On Call.* 5(5):30–31. Available at http://www.healthliteracy.com/using-stories. Accessed April 6, 2011.

Osborne H. 2008. In Other Words . . . Tools of Change: Telling and Listening to Stories. *On Call.* Available at http://www.healthliteracy.com/telling-stories. Accessed February 9, 2011.

Quesenbery W, Brooks K. 2010. *Storytelling for User Experience.* Brooklyn, NY: Rosenfeld Media.

SOURCES TO LEARN MORE

Charon R. 2004. Narrative and Medicine. *New England Journal of Medicine.* 350(9):862–864.

Charon R. 2006. *Narrative Medicine: Honoring the Stories of Illness.* New York: Oxford University Press.

Denning S. 2004, May. Telling Tales. *Harvard Business Review.* Cambridge, MA: Harvard Business School Publishing.

Denning S. 2005. *The Leader's Guide to Storytelling: Mastering the Art and Discipline of Business Narrative.* San Francisco: Jossey-Bass.

Greenhalgh T, Collard A, Begum N. 2005. Sharing Stories: Complex Intervention for Diabetes Education in Minority Ethnic Groups Who Do Not Speak English. *British Medical Journal.* 330:628.

Healing Story Alliance, http://www.healingstory.org/home.html.

Houston TK, Allison JJ, Sussman M, Horn W, Holt CL, Trobaugh J, et al. 2011. Culturally Appropriate Storytelling to Improve Blood Pressure. *Annals of Internal Medicine.* 154(2):77–84.

International Storytelling Center, http://www.storytellingcenter.net/.

Kreuter MW, Holmes K, Alcaraz K, Kalesan B, Rath S, Richert M., et al. 2010. Comparing Narrative and Informational Videos to Increase Mammography in Low-Income African American Women. *Patient Education and Counseling.* 8(S1):S6–S14.

LANES (League for the Advancement of New England Storytelling), http://www.lanes.org/.

National Storytelling Network, http://www.storynet.org.

Newman TB. 2003. The Power of Stories over Statistics. *British Medical Journal.* 327:1424–1427.

Osborne H (host). 2010, May 11. Folktales as Tools for Healing [audio podcast]. *Health Literacy Out Loud,* no. 37. Available at http://www.healthliteracy.com/hlol-folktales. Accessed February 9, 2011.

Teaching and Learning

STARTING POINTS

All healthcare encounters are opportunities for providers to teach, exchange knowledge, and engage in mutual learning with patients. This includes teaching patients about their diagnoses and treatment options. It also includes learning about patients' symptoms, priorities, and choices.

Health teaching and learning can happen informally, as when chatting with patients just before procedures and tests, or more formally in structured educational situations. Here are some examples:

- *One-to-one teaching.* This traditionally has referred to the dyad of one healthcare professional and one patient. But today, there may be more people involved, such as health care team members and the patient's family members, caregiver, or perhaps an interpreter.
- *Health education classes.* These are usually led by a health professional and structured with a formal curriculum and clear-cut goals. Classes may focus on specific topics such as diseases and medical procedures or on more general themes like wellness and health promotion.
- *Support and self-help groups.* Usually led by a patient or consumer, these types of groups tend to be fairly informal with built-in flexibility to accommodate participants' specific needs and interests.
- *Group visits.* This relatively new model of care combines group teaching and interaction with elements of an individual patient visit such as the collection of vital signs, history taking, and physical exam (for details on this model, see Jaber, Braksmajer, & Trilling 2006).

Teaching about health is challenging for many reasons. Instructions may be complicated and explained in unfamiliar words and with lots of numbers. People may have limited literacy or language skills, cognitive changes, or other learning barriers. And when patients are overwhelmed with new diagnoses or are scared, sick, and in pain, they likely are not at their learning best. Below are some ways to teach, learn, and help patients take action.

STRATEGIES, IDEAS, AND SUGGESTIONS

Here are some strategies you might put into practice (Osborne 2002, January; 2002, June; 2002, July/August; 2007, June 26; 2009, May 26):

Appreciate that people learn in many ways. Some people are auditory learners and learn best when listening to lectures or hearing instructions read aloud. Others are visual learners who understand by looking at pictures or reading books. And still others are kinesthetic learners who absorb information when touching objects or doing activities. Often, people have more than one learning style and learn best through a combination of ways.

It often helps to use a variety of teaching strategies. For instance, when teaching someone newly diagnosed with asthma, you might talk with her about the condition (auditory), show her a model of a lung and let her practice using an inhaler (kinesthetic), and give her booklets to read when she is at home (visual).

Time your teaching for when patients are ready to learn. The timing of your teaching is often as important as its content, for patients may be unable to learn when they are distracted or uncomfortable. Take your cues from patients about how much information to present in each session. For example, if a person seems to "tune out" after a short while, consider scheduling a follow-up meeting to continue teaching later on.

Encourage patients to be active learners. People learn best when they are actively involved in the learning process, not just passive recipients of information. Ask patients what they want to learn and, together, set the teaching agenda. Make sure that you allow plenty of opportunities for interaction with sufficient time for patients to ask questions and raise concerns. And, of course, provide lists of print and non-print resources for people who want to learn more.

Give a "heads up" about the topics you plan to discuss. Talk about topics one at a time, and make sure that patients understand each key point before moving to the next. At the end of teaching sessions, summarize main ideas and topics. Be consistent; use the same terminology and demonstrate techniques the same way each time.

Build on familiar information, tying new learning to old. For example, instead of talking abstractly about proper body mechanics, you might instead teach a young mother how to pick up a baby without straining her back. Make sure, as well, to find out what patients already know or believe to be true. Sometimes you need to clarify misconceptions and correct misunderstandings before introducing new information.

Explain instructions in plain language. This includes defining unfamiliar, but essential, words and giving people examples to help them understand. For instance, instead of just instructing patients to "lift no more than five pounds," let them know that five pounds is the same weight as a bag of flour. As well, clarify instructions like "take pills twice daily." While you might mean "take one pill in the morning and one at night," patients might assume they can take two pills at the same time. (Read more in "Plain Language," starting on page 157.)

Prioritize "need to know" survival information. In the hurried environment of health care, we need to make sure every teachable moment is used effectively, says Sandra Cornett, PhD, RN, who is the Director of AHEC Clear Health Communication Program at Ohio State University. To figure out what is most important, Cornett recommends prioritizing (1) actions patients need for survival, (2) actions that are the easiest for patients to change or do, and (3) resources available to help patients take those actions. (Cornett 2011)

Watch for cues that you are going either too fast or too slow. A good way is by observing whether people look "glazed over" or their body language indicates they are bored. You can also ask people if you are teaching at a good pace. This is admittedly easier to do when meeting one to one. But, even when teaching a group, you can check the pace by stopping periodically and giving people the opportunity to ask questions and practice or demonstrate what they are learning. Encourage them to also let you know if you are speaking too softly or if printed information is too small to see or hard to understand.

Confirm understanding. The goal of all learning and teaching is knowledge. Make sure that people truly understand and can make use of the information you are presenting. Stop periodically and make sure that patients are keeping up with you. You can do this by asking people to tell you, in their own words, that they understand what you are saying or show you how they will accomplish skills you just taught. As knowledge is a two-way process, make sure to confirm that you understand what patients are teaching you, too.

Stories from Practice: Helping Patients Take Action

The goal of most health care teaching is for patients to take needed actions, such as changing activity and dietary habits. Rather than dictating what to do, providers can help by acting as coaches—helping patients think of, select, and accomplish doable actions. Terry Davis, PhD, is a leading health literacy researcher. In a *Health Literacy Out Loud Podcast*, she spoke about this process, referring to it as "Baby Steps."

Davis tells about a woman who needed to lose 25 pounds. To this woman, 25 pounds felt like an unobtainable goal. The woman's everyday routine was to buy fast food on her way home from work. With coaching from her doctor, the woman chose a "baby step" (small, achievable goal) of cooking dinner one night a week rather than buying fast food. The woman lost some weight as a result. She then increased the goal to cooking dinner at home three or four nights each week. And yes, this woman did eventually lose 25 pounds.

Davis credits this success to the baby step process. "The patient is in charge. It is easily doable, empowering, boosts confidence, and helps change behaviors one step at a time."

Source: Osborne (2009, May 26).

 Knowledge is a two-way process. Make sure that patients truly understand and can use the information you are presenting. Make sure to also confirm that you understand what others are teaching you, too.

CITATIONS

Cornett S. 2011. Personal communication.

Jaber R, Braksmajer A, Trilling J. 2006. Group Visits for Chronic Illness Care: Models, Benefits and Challenges. *Family Practice Management.* 13(1):37–40.

Osborne H. 2002, January. In Other Words . . . Making the Match . . . Choosing Patient Education Materials. *On Call.* Available at http://www.healthliteracy.com/choosing-patient-education-materials. Accessed February 14, 2011.

Osborne H. 2002, June. In Other Words . . . Getting Formal . . . Educating Patients in a Classroom Setting. *On Call.* Available at http://www.healthliteracy.com/ classroom-setting. Accessed February 14, 2011.

Osborne H. 2002, July/August. In Other Words . . . Getting Formal . . . Finding the Teaching Tools You Need at a Price Your Organization Can Afford. *On Call.* Available at http://www.healthliteracy.com/teaching-tools. Accessed February 14, 2011.

Osborne H. 2007, June 26. In Other Words . . . How to Help Patients Manage Their Action Planning. *On Call.* Available at http://www.healthliteracy.com/action-planning. Accessed August 16, 2010.

Osborne H (host). 2009, May 26. Terry Davis Talks About "Baby Steps" (Action Planning) [audio podcast]. *Health Literacy Out Loud,* no. 16. Available at http://www.healthliteracy.com/hlol-action-planning. Accessed February 14, 2011.

SOURCES TO LEARN MORE

American College of Physicians (ACP) Foundation. 2007. *Living with Diabetes: An Everyday Guide for You and Your Family.* Copies available from http://foundation.acponline.org/hl/diabguide.htm. Accessed February 14, 2011.

Angelmar R, Berman PC. 2007. *Patient Empowerment and Efficient Health Outcomes.* Financing Sustainable Healthcare in Europe: New Approaches for New Outcomes. Available at http://www.drmed.org/javne_datoteke/novice/datoteke/10483-Report_3.pdf. Accessed July 11, 2011.

Bodenheimer T. 2008. Coordinating Care: A Perilous Journey Through the Health Care System. *New England Journal of Medicine.* 358(10):1064–1071.

Bodenheimer T, Davis C, Holman H. 2007. Helping Patients Adopt Healthier Behaviors. *Clinical Diabetes.* 25(2):66–70.

Cordasco KM, Asch SM, Bell DS, Guterman JJ, Gross-Schulman S, Ramer L, et al. 2009. A Low-Literacy Medication Education Tool for Safety-Net Hospital Patients. *American Journal of Preventive Medicine.* 37(6, Suppl. 1):S209–S216.

DeWalt DA, Davis TC, Wallace AS, Seligman HK, Bryant-Shilliday B, Arnold CL, et al. 2009. Goal Setting in Diabetes Self-Management: Taking the Baby Steps to Success. *Patient Education and Counseling.* 77(2):218–223.

Dickinson D, Raynor DKT. 2003. Ask the Patients—They May Want to Know More Than You Think. *British Medical Journal.* 327(7419):861. Available at http://www.ncbi.nlm.nih.gov/pmc/articles/PMC214093/. Accessed February 14, 2011.

Handley M, MacGregor K, Schillinger D, Sharifi C, Wong S, Bodenheimer T. 2006. Using Action Plans to Help Primary Care Patients Adopt Healthy Behaviors: A Descriptive Study. *Journal of the American Board of Family Medicine.* 19(3): 224–231.

Knowles MS. 1988. *The Modern Practice of Adult Education: From Pedagogy to Andragogy.* Rev. ed. Englewood Cliffs, NJ: Cambridge Adult Education.

Knowles MS. 1990. *The Adult Learner: A Neglected Species.* 4th ed. Houston, TX: Gulf Publishing.

Kripalani S, Robertson R, Love-Ghaffari MH, Henderson LE, Praska J, Strawder A, et al. 2007. Development of an Illustrated Medication Schedule as a Low-Literacy Patient Education Tool. *Patient Education and Counseling.* 66(3):368–377.

London F. 2010. *No Time to Teach: The Essence of Patient and Family Education for Health Care Providers.* 2nd ed. Atlanta, GA: Pritchett & Hull.

Lorig K. 2006. Action Planning: A Call to Action. *Journal of the American Board of Family Medicine.* 19(3):324–325.

Seligman HK, Wallace AS, DeWalt DA, Schillinger D, Arnold CL, Shilliday BB, et al. 2007. Facilitating Behavior Change with Low-Literacy Patient Education Materials. *American Journal of Health Behavior* 31(Suppl.):S69–S78.

Wallace AS, Seligman HK, Davis TC, Schillinger D, Arnold CL, Bryant-Shilliday B, et al. 2009. Literacy-Appropriate Educational Materials and Brief Counseling Improve Diabetes Self-Management. *Patient Education and Counseling.* 75(3):328–333.

Technology: Audio Podcasts

STARTING POINTS

The technical definition of podcasts is that they are digital media files distributed over the Internet. A more descriptive explanation is that podcasts are like radio shows with informational or entertaining audio content. What distinguishes the two is that listeners can choose when, where, and how to hear podcasts.

To listen, start by finding the file you want on the Internet—the iTunes store (http://www.apple.com/itunes/) is a great resource. Once you download the iTunes program file, you can listen directly from your computer or use it to add audio files to your cell phone, iPod, or other MP3 device. When you find podcasts that you especially like, see if there is a way to subscribe. This means that you automatically get the latest files. I am such a fan of podcasts that they are part of my daily routine. In fact, I cannot imagine going on my morning walk without listening to them.

Podcasts offer more opportunities than just listening. You can produce content as well. That's what I have been doing with my ongoing series, *Health Literacy Out Loud*. These podcasts are a way for health literacy advocates everywhere to hear and learn from those "in the know" about the topic. Below is information about producing podcasts. You can listen and learn more about *Health Literacy Out Loud* podcasts at www .healthliteracyoutloud.com.

Strategies, Ideas, and Suggestions

Here are some ideas to consider (Osborne & Weiss 2009):

Weigh the benefits and risks of podcasting. Benefits of podcasting include positioning yourself as an expert, distinguishing yourself from competitors, raising your online visibility, and expanding your set of communication skills. But podcasting also brings risks and costs, including committing time and money, as well as the uncertainty of trying something new.

Stories from Practice: Producing Audio Podcasts

Adam Weiss edits all of Helen Osborne's *Health Literacy Out Loud* podcasts. In a podcast about podcasting, Weiss spoke about how this technology can amplify the health literacy message. "Podcasts are a way to learn about health literacy at a convenient time and place," he explains. "This suits health professionals as they can fit the learning into their everyday routine."

Weiss compares podcasts to the radio. "On the radio, health literacy is a topic that people may hear about only once every few weeks, or months," he says. "With a podcast you can present in-depth information that a listener wouldn't otherwise get. No matter how good you are, radio stations are unlikely to create a 'Health Literacy Channel' unless you create one with a podcast."

And that's exactly what Helen Osborne did—with help from Adam Weiss, of course.

Source: Osborne (2010, August 1).

Choose a podcast format. The three most common formats are:

- **Highly produced radio shows.** This is when several segments are recorded "in the field" and later mixed together in a sound studio. An example is Chicago Public Radio's *This American Life with Ira Glass* (http://www.thisamericanlife.org/podcast/).
- **Lecture format.** This is just one person talking. Honestly, these are often less than compelling to listen to. An example of a lecture format done well is the BBC's *From Our Own Correspondent* (http://www.bbc .co.uk/podcasts/series/fooc/).

- **Interview.** To do an interview show well you need to be an excellent questioner, listener, and committed to making guests shine more than you. *Health Literacy Out Loud* is an example of an interview show.

Decide about time. This includes the length of each edited podcast and frequency of new episodes. Twenty minutes is a good upper limit for most podcasts, and five minutes is usually the lower limit. The ideal is to podcast at least once or twice a month, as listeners will come to expect new and timely information.

Acquire needed technology. You can record podcasts in person or over the phone. To record podcasts in person, you need a good-quality digital recorder. It helps to also have a handheld microphone to better control the conversation. To record podcasts over the phone (as I usually do), you need:

- *Skype.* This computer-based program (available at www.skype.com) is a way to make phone calls over the Internet. The sound quality for podcasts is excellent so long as you use a good microphone and the other person talks on a corded landline, not Skype. An added benefit is that there is no or minimal cost for most calls.
- *Microphone.* The audio quality is far better when you use a good microphone, not just the one in your computer. Make sure to plug in the microphone before turning on Skype so the computer knows which to use.
- *Headset.* You need to listen while recording. The best way to do this is with a good-quality headset.
- *Software to save recorded calls.* You'll need additional software to save these recorded calls. Options include Call Burner for the PC (www .callburner.com) and Call Recorder for the Macintosh (http://www .ecamm.com/mac/callrecorder/).

Edit the podcast. To me, it is important to produce a professional-sounding podcast. That's why I work with an experienced audio editor. If you edit the podcasts yourself, you will need a software program to cut up and rearrange the audio segments. There are several free or inexpensive options for both the PC and Macintosh.

Make the podcast available to others. The simplest way is by making an MP3 file and posting it to a blog, such as WordPress (www.wordpress.org).

You can also make the podcast available to millions of potential listeners by posting it on iTunes. Consider also offering a written transcript so that your podcast is accessible to those who are Deaf, hard of hearing, or want a printed version of the audio conversation.

 I am such a fan of podcasts that they are part of my daily routine. In fact, I cannot imagine going on my morning walk without listening to them.

CITATIONS

Osborne H, Weiss A. 2009. *Podcasting Guide: A Little About Technology, A Lot About Getting Started with Audio Interviews* Available at http://healthliteracy.com/ podcasting-guide. Accessed April 7, 2011.

Osborne H (host). 2010, August 1. Adam Weiss Talks About Podcasting [audio podcast]. *Health Literacy Out Loud,* no. 1. Available at http://healthliteracy.com/ hlol-podcasting. Accessed August 1, 2010.

SOURCES TO LEARN MORE

Abel J, Glass I. 1999. *Radio: An Illustrated Guide.* Chicago: WBEZ Alliance.

Gross T. 2005. *All I Did Was Ask: Conversations with Writers, Actors, Musicians, and Artists.* New York: Hyperion.

Hobson EH, Haines SL, Van Amburgh JA. 2010. Meeting the Challenge of Public Health Information Delivery in the Digital Age. *Journal of the American Pharmacists Association.* 50(2):214–217.

Osborne H (host). 2011, July 12. Using the Internet for Health [audio podcast]. Health Literacy Out Loud no. 62. Available at http://healthliteracy.com/ hlol-pew. Accessed July 12, 2011.

Technology: Blogs and Other Social Media

STARTING POINTS

Social media is as significant a milestone in communication as the invention of the printing press, radio, and television, some technology experts believe. Social media is being used in all aspects of our lives, including health communication.

Pamela Katz Ressler, RN, MS, HN-BC, is president and founder of Stress Resources, LLC, based in Massachusetts. She and I spoke several times, including on a *Health Literacy Out Loud* podcast, about the benefits of blogging and other social media within a healthcare context. Ressler says that one compelling reason to use these media is that they reach traditionally underserved populations. She cites studies showing that two new populations are "jumping online." They are (1) non-college-educated 18- to 30-year-olds who are connecting via mobile phones, rather than computers, and (2) older adults (60 years old and over) who are becoming more interested in and comfortable with technology, especially computers. Certainly, these populations are ones that health professionals want to reach, and teach (Osborne 2011, February 15).

Stories from Practice: Social Media Is Like a Food Pyramid

Lee Aase works in the communications department at Mayo Clinic in Rochester, Minnesota. He also has his own business, SMUG (Social Media University Global; http://social-media-university-global.org/), and has dubbed himself its chancellor. I interviewed Aase for a *Health Literacy Out Loud* podcast. He equated social media to a food pyramid:

- **Micro-blogging is the base.** Aase is referring primarily to "tweets," which are very short Twitter messages of no more than 140 characters, including spaces. He recommends many daily "portions" of micro-blogging. These include tweeting and re-tweeting (forwarding) messages with interesting news and links.
- **Social networking is the next level.** It includes networking forums and sites such as Facebook and LinkedIn. To Aase, social networking enables contact with many more friends and colleagues than would be possible in real life.
- **Multimedia makes up the third level.** It includes audio podcasts and videos. Aase says that this type of multimedia offers more in-depth content than either of the levels below. But multimedia does require some special equipment and a degree of technical savvy.
- **Blogs are at the pyramid's peak.** The benefit of blogs is that they provide in-depth information on a narrow topic. Aase sees a link between blogs and traditional journalism. "Be the media, don't just pitch the media," he says.

Source: Osborne (2010, March 19).

STRATEGIES, IDEAS, AND SUGGESTIONS

Here are some social media strategies you may find useful (Osborne 2011, February 15; Ressler 2010):

Get your social media feet wet, so to speak. We all have to start somewhere when it comes to social media. The Internet is filled with resources to learn about and get started with Twitter, Facebook, blogs, and other types of social media. If you are reluctant to participate, you might begin by looking at examples. You can easily find them by doing a search with key words like "patient blogs." Pay close attention to what people write about and how often they post (add) new content. Then, at some point, muster your courage and try these tools yourself. Really, social media is not as difficult as you might first fear.

Appreciate the value of social media to you and your patients. Here are two examples:

- *Social media as an adjunct to patient education.* You can use social media to inform and teach, such as tweeting about the latest health news or posting up-to-date research about a certain disease or condition. One example is the Mayo Clinic blogs in which experts post information about a range of health topics (http://www.mayoclinic.com/health/blogs/BlogIndex).
- *Patient blogs as an expression of illness.* Ressler says that blogs offer tremendous potential for helping patients feel less alone and more in control of an illness or caregiving situation. Patients often write about experiences from their first diagnosis to finding a "new normal" in their lives. An example is the blog from Dana Jennings on the *New York Times* Web site (http://well.blogs.nytimes.com/tag/jennings/).

Address concerns. Admittedly, social media brings some very real concerns. They include:

- *Privacy.* Ressler recommends that healthcare professionals create clear boundaries between their public and private use of social media. This can be using different names or identifiers and setting privacy controls as to whether you want information shared publicly (so everyone can see) or privately (available only to certain people).
- *Payment.* As yet, there is little to no third-party reimbursement for the extra time you spend communicating through social media. This may be a reason to limit the extent to which you communicate with patients online.
- *Time.* Yes, social media takes time. Just like with other competing demands, you need to budget how much time you can reasonably allot. For some, social media is so appealing and intriguing that hours can go by without much notice.

> **Stories from Practice: Social Media Creates Personal Connections**
>
> Pam Ressler's interest in social media began as a mom, not as a nurse. In 2001, her 14-year-old son Nick was hospitalized with advanced cancer. While blogs and social media hadn't yet been invented, Nick liked staying in touch with his school friends by IM (instant messaging—like text messages today). "Nick wanted to be a kid without his cancer diagnosis in the forefront," says Ressler. By IM-ing with his friends, she says that Nick could maintain a sense of normalcy despite his incredibly difficult situation.
>
> Sadly, Nick died. But his enthusiasm for connecting through technology lives on. Ressler sees tremendous potential for social media to allow people, no matter their diagnoses or limitations, to create incredible and personal connections in age-appropriate, no-hassle ways.
>
> *Source:* Ressler (2010). You can read Ressler's blog at http://pamressler.blogspot.com

 Social media is as significant a milestone in communication as the invention of the printing press, radio, and television, some technology experts believe.

CITATIONS

Osborne H (host). 2010, March 19. Social Media and Health Literacy [audio podcast]. *Health Literacy Out Loud*, no. 33. Available at http://www.healthliteracy.com/hlol-social-media. Accessed October 12, 2010.

Osborne H (host). 2011, February 15. Blogging to Communicate the Experience of Illness [audio podcast]. *Health Literacy Out Loud*, no. 53. Available at http://www.healthliteracy.com/hlol-blogging. Accessed February 17, 2011.

Ressler P. 2010. Personal communication.

SOURCES TO LEARN MORE

Increasing Stress Resilience and Balance in Health Care, Education, Work and Life [blog]. Available at http://pamressler.blogspot.com/.

Keckley PH, Hoffmann M. 2010. *Issue Brief: Social Networks in HealthCare: Communication, Collaboration, and Insights*. The Deloitte Center for Health

Solutions. Available at https://www.deloitte.com/view/en_US/us/industries/ US-federal-government/center-for-health-solutions/disruptive-innovations/ 2fbc755f3c1b9210VgnVCM100000ba42f00aRCRD.htm. Accessed February 16, 2011.

Mearian L. 2010, May 20. E-health and Web 2.0: The Doctor Will Tweet You Now. *Computerworld*. Available at http://hbr.org/2004/05/telling-tales/ar/1. Accessed August 15, 2011.

Technology: Email and Text Messaging

STARTING POINTS

Ready or not, email and text messaging are increasingly being used to communicate health information. The Pew Internet & American Life Project provides a wealth of up-to-date data about the growing use of broadband, mobile, and other technology important in our daily lives (Pew Internet 2010).

STRATEGIES, IDEAS, AND SUGGESTIONS

Here are some ideas about using email and text messaging in practice (Osborne 2003; 2008):

Take advantage of the benefits of using email in healthcare settings. People may respond at their convenience, messages can be printed and saved, and hyperlinks can be added so people need only to click for more information. But email also brings concerns about privacy and security. For instance, people who share computers can sometimes access messages intended for others, and employers can legally read messages their employees send from work. Many patients and providers feel that the benefits of email outweigh its drawbacks.

Stories from Practice: Email

Ann lives about three hours away from her primary care doctor. While mowing her lawn, she was bitten on her finger by a wasp. Ann knew it wasn't an emergency but was concerned that her finger was infected when it swelled up and turned a fierce-looking red. So she emailed her doctor and attached digital photos of her finger.

Seeing this picture, the doctor felt that Ann's reaction was only inflammatory and didn't require emergency treatment. He recommended she apply ice, elevate her hand, and email him again in 48 hours. He also wrote in his email reply that Ann should go to a local emergency department if her symptoms worsened. Two days later, Ann emailed back, "You were right. The bite already subsided."

Source: Osborne (2003).

- *Make it clear that email is not to be used for medical emergencies.* Patients need to fully understand that email is not to be used for emergencies. There is no guarantee that providers will see messages quickly enough, nor is there any assurance that patients will read responses in time to take immediate action. While in the example above, Ann was sure that her situation did not require immediate attention, in other instances patients may not know what constitutes an emergency. As part of good clinical practice, talk with patients about health problems that need attention right away.
- *Use plain language.* Make sure your email messages are easy to read. This means using plain-language principles such as common one- and two-syllable words, short sentences with no more than 15 words, and short paragraphs with only two or three sentences. These principles are even more important when replying to patient's messages that have a lot of spelling, punctuation, and vocabulary errors—indications the writer may have problems with literacy or language.
- *Replying to messages.* Let patients know when to expect replies from you—such as within 24 hours, or one to two days. In addition, create an "auto responder" that automatically notifies patients when you receive their message. In this automated reply, include a phone number where patients can call for more immediate assistance.

- *Consider the most appropriate way to respond.* Just because patients send you email messages doesn't mean you need to reply the same way. For example, you likely will not want to use email when conveying bad news or discussing complex treatment options. Instead, you might email to arrange a follow-up phone or in-person appointment to talk more about these issues.

Use text messaging. Text messaging is being adopted as a helpful, timely, non-intrusive communication tool. All people have to do is pick up the phone and the message is there. Increasingly, hospitals and clinics and other health-related organizations are using text messages to teach about health.

Stories from Practice: Text Messaging

In 2007, at a clinic for teenagers with asthma at the Children's Hospital Medical Center in Cincinnati, Ohio, hospital staff noticed that teens were often text messaging their friends and parents. This was happening whether they were getting blood drawn, getting a shot, or even talking with doctors.

Several teens with asthma were on the hospital's Teen Advisory Board. Since they were texting one another even in the same room, someone suggested using the technology for medication reminders. The teens wholeheartedly supported the idea and volunteered to help develop a system for doing so.

About 20 teens with asthma (ages 12 to 21) received a text reminder message once or twice a day. The frequency depended on how often they needed medication. The message contained no additional information about which medicine to take or who sent the message since the teens already knew these things. They also knew that the message was about taking routine "controller" medications to prevent asthma attacks, and not about "rescue" medications needed only when attacks occur.

Source: Osborne (2008).

The following tips about text messaging are from experiences at the Children's Hospital Medical Center in Cincinnati, Ohio (see Stories from Practice: Text Messaging). While this project lasted just a year, studies are under way to evaluate the long-term benefit of texting health messages (Munafo 2011).

- *Offer the option of text messaging.* Whether teens are newly diagnosed or have been dealing with asthma for many years, clinicians are usually the ones to initiate a discussion about text message medication reminders. More often than not, teens and their parents respond well when clinicians say, "We have this program that can help you remember to take medications. If you're interested, we can start right away."
- *Obtain consent.* At the hospital in Cincinnati, teens were given a simple one-page form specifying that they will receive a text message (either once or twice a day) and agree to pay any phone-related charges that may accrue. For teens under 18, their parents must also agree. For many teens, there is no additional cost if their cell phone plan includes unlimited text messaging.
- *Designate someone to send daily messages.* Initially, the program started with a small trial in which the "Parent Coordinator" sent messages at pre-determined times to all the teens. Unlike email, where people can often see who else is receiving the same message, there is no concern about privacy. Each teen reads only the message that comes to his or her phone.
- *Make the message clear, but brief.* The Teen Advisory Board talked about how to word the reminder message. They cautioned adults not to be cool and use slang or text shorthand. They wanted all words spelled out so as not to be confusing. So the message uses terms like "forget," not "4get." Sometimes there is a little something extra, such as a friendly or timely "Have a great day" or "Happy Halloween."

 Just because patients send you email messages doesn't mean you need to reply the same way. For example, you likely will not want to use email when conveying bad news or discussing complex treatment options.

CITATIONS

Munafo J. 2011. Personal communication.

Osborne H. 2003. In Other Words . . . Communicating Electronically with Patients. *On Call.* 6(8):16–17. Available at http://healthliteracy.com/communicating-electronically. Accessed February 18, 2011.

Osborne H. 2008, September 18. In Other Words . . . Using Text Messages to Improve Medication Adherence. *On Call.* Available at http://www.healthliteracy.com/text-messages. Accessed February 18, 2011.

Pew Internet. Trend Data. December 2010 Survey. Available at http://www.pewinternet.org/Static-Pages/Trend-Data/Online-Activites-Total.aspx. Accessed July 18, 2011.

SOURCES TO LEARN MORE

American Medical Association. 2002. *Guidelines for Physician-Patient Electronic Communications.* Available at http://www.ama-assn.org/ama/pub/about-ama/ our-people/member-groups-sections/young-physicians-section/advocacy-resources/guidelines-physician-patient-electronic-communications.shtml. Accessed February 18, 2011.

Barclay L. 2007, October 3. Patient-Physician Email Communication May Be Effective. *Medscape Medical News.* Available at http://www.medscape.org/ viewarticle/563678. Accessed February 18, 2011.

Britto MT, DeVellis RF, Hornung RW, DeFriese GH, Atherton HD, Slap GB. 2004. Health Care Preferences and Priorities of Adolescents with Chronic Illnesses. *Pediatrics.* 114(5):1272–1280.

Fox S. 2010, September 13. *The Power of Mobile.* Prepared for Mayo Transform 2010: Thinking Differently About Health Care. Available at http://e-patients.net/ archives/2010/09/the-power-of-mobile.html. Accessed February 18, 2011.

HealthyEmail. A source for HealthyEmail tools, including sample consent forms. Available at http://www.healthyemail.org/toolkit.php.

Osborne H (host). 2011, April 26. Texting Important Health Messages [audio podcast]. *Health Literacy Out Loud,* no. 56. Available at http://healthliteracy .com/hlol-texting. Accessed April 26, 2011.

Osborne H (host). 2011, July 12. Using the Internet for Health [audio podcast]. *Health Literacy Out Loud* no. 62. Available at http://healthliteracy.com/hlol-pew. Accessed July 12, 2011.

Text4Baby. Available at http://text4baby.org.

Technology:
Interactive Multimedia

STARTING POINTS

Technology allows us to do amazing things, including simulating interactions that might actually occur between patients and their healthcare providers. This is accomplished thanks to interactive technology using "multi-path" or "branching" logic, which customizes information based on input from each user. Beyond interactivity, this type of technology also allows for multimedia so you can present information in text, animation, illustrations, and the spoken word.

Given the rapid development of new technology, it is likely that there will be numerous options for interactive media in patient education. This chapter is a place to start.

STRATEGIES, IDEAS, AND SUGGESTIONS

Here are some suggestions to consider (Osborne 2004; 2010, September 14):

Research what people are saying about the subject. When creating a new interactive product or Web site, include not only evidence-based research but also information from real people. Research can include focus groups, interviews, and "eavesdropping" on public blogs and chat rooms. Listen carefully to how people describe their needs, challenges, and barriers and then, as appropriate, use these words and examples in your project.

> ### Stories from Practice: Interactive "Conversations" from Healthwise
>
> Healthwise, a nonprofit health communications company based in Boise, Idaho, has developed several interactive multimedia "Conversations" on a range of health and wellness topics. These simulated interactions respond in a personal way depending on how users answer dozens of questions. For example, in a Healthwise Conversation about "Dealing with Low Back Pain," users are asked:
>
> - Do you know what caused the pain?
> - Was the pain a result of an accident or serious injury?
> - How long have you been in pain?
> - What treatments have you already tried?
>
> Based on the user's response from a list of options, an empathetic narrator teaches about this condition. As indicated, the narrator also highlights self-management strategies for time, medication, and activity. Multimedia helps engage users in this Conversation. One way is with the ongoing metaphor "The back is like a bridge." This metaphor is not only spoken but also used graphically to show how low back pain is like when trusses or cables of a bridge break down.
>
> Healthwise's Conversations have been extensively tested. User feedback is overwhelmingly positive, with people saying that these interactive Conversations help them better understand their condition and increase confidence about ways to manage it.
>
> *Source:* Healthwise (2009; 2010).

Develop your project with a team. Ideally, team members will include subject matter experts, plain language writers, designers, animators, usability testers, and "end users" representing the intended audience. For instance, when Healthwise created its interactive product about preventing falls in the elderly, they talked with someone who teaches a falls-prevention class as well as members of the local senior center.

Use plain language. This means using words that are clear, simple, common, and consistent throughout. For instance, if you are teaching about low back pain, then consistently refer to it this way rather than also saying "spinal problems."

Teach in the many ways that people learn. Interactive multimedia is an ideal format for meeting the varied needs of learners. For instance, visual learners may learn best by watching an animation or looking at an anatomic drawing. Auditory learners might prefer listening to the spoken word. And those who learn best by reading can print out a written summary. Karen Baker, Senior Vice President of Healthwise, says that when you present information in an engaging, multimodal way, "there is a better chance that people will remember and learn" (Osborne 2010, September 14).

As possible, tailor information to your audience. Learn as much as you can about the intended audience. And then, if possible, tailor content to their experiences and interests. For instance, when creating an interactive Web site about nutrition for an audience of people from Haiti, you could include traditional Haitian foods such as rice, beans, and chicken.

Honor the preferences of your users. Do your users appreciate some humor about this condition? Or do they feel that humor means that their problems are not being taken seriously? Learn what your users need, want, and appreciate by asking about humor, illustrations, and metaphors in user testing.

Make sure your product is accessible to all (508 Compliant). The U.S. Rehabilitation Act of 1973 (referred to as "Section 508 Laws") requires federal agencies to make their electronic and information technology accessible to people with disabilities. This law includes text captioning for the audio, audio descriptions for the visuals, and navigation options using keyboard controls rather than a computer mouse. Learn more at Section508 .gov (http://www.section508.gov).

 Beyond interactivity, multimedia technology allows you to present information in text, animation, illustrations, and the spoken word. 99

Citations

Healthwise. 2009. *Conversation on Dealing With Low Back Pain.* Available at http://www.healthwise.org/backconversation. Accessed July 30, 2010.

Healthwise. 2010. Personal communication.

Osborne H. 2004, January/February. In Other Words . . . Teaching with Touchscreen Technology. *On Call.* Available at http://www.healthliteracy.com/touchscreen-technology. Accessed July 30, 2010.

Osborne H (host). 2010, September 14. Interactive Multimedia in Health Education [audio podcast]. *Health Literacy Out Loud,* no. 45. Available at http://healthliteracy.com/hlol-interactive-multimedia. Accessed February 14, 2011.

Sources to Learn More

Kemper DW, Del Fiol G, Hall LK, Myers S, Gutierrez J. 2010. *Getting Patients to Meaningful Use: Using the HL7 Infobutton Standard for Information Prescriptions.* Prepared for Healthwise, Incorporated. Available at http://www.healthwise .org/Insights.aspx. Accessed July 28, 2010.

Wofford JL, Currin D, Michielutte R, Wofford MM. 2001. The Multimedia Computer for Low-Literacy Patient Education: A Pilot Project of Cancer Risk Perceptions. *Medscape General Medicine.* 3(2).

Universal Design
in Communication

STARTING POINTS

Universal design describes a concept of designing products, environments, and communications that not only considers the specific needs of people with disabilities, but also takes into account the more universal changes that everyone faces as they age. Curb cuts on sidewalks are an example of universal design. They not only help people in wheelchairs but also are valued by parents with baby strollers and travelers with wheeled suitcases.

Likewise in health communications, universal design can be helpful to all. This includes easy-to-read brochures and easy-to-use Web sites that most everyone can see, understand, and use. "If a design works well for a person with a disability, it probably works better for everybody," says Valerie Fletcher, Executive Director of the Institute for Human Centered Design in Boston (Osborne 2001, January).

STRATEGIES, IDEAS, AND SUGGESTIONS

Here are some strategies you may find useful (Osborne 2001; 2010, October 5):

Presume that people do not have full function. Rather than trying to figure out who has what limitation, focus instead on communicating clearly with everyone. Make it a habit to incorporate principles of universal design in all forms of communication, whether it is in person, in print, or on the Web.

Stories from Practice: Universal Design as a Framework to Communicate with Everyone

In a *Health Literacy Out Loud* podcast, Valerie Fletcher spoke about the functional limitations that people face as they live longer or survive serious illnesses and accidents. Rather than thinking of these as disabilities or deficits, Fletcher describes them as an "incredible diversity of abilities."

But such diverse abilities are not necessarily obvious or even extraordinary. In a routine healthcare visit, for example, a patient with a slight hearing loss might miss key points of what the doctor is saying. And it's quite possible that neither the doctor nor the patient is aware that this is happening.

Universal design is a framework to communicate clearly with everyone, not just those who have obvious or identified needs. In the example above, this means that the doctor would communicate in redundant ways—communicating the message by speaking clearly, using simply written materials, demonstrating on models, and illustrating with visuals.

Source: Osborne (2010, October 5).

Use redundant communication. This means conveying the same message in multiple ways. For instance, when explaining to a patient why it's good to get a flu shot, you can discuss it, distribute a one-page flyer, suggest relevant Web sites, and provide a phone number that people can call to learn more.

Consider the "built environment." Good communication depends on not only what we say or do but also the environment in which we meet with others. Look critically at where you work.

- Is the navigation intuitive? This means that outsiders can quickly figure out where to go. If it's not intuitive, then find ways to make navigation easier, such as having a staffed "help desk" and not just written signs.
- Pay attention to acoustics. Is there a noisy air conditioner or heater in rooms where you meet with patients? If so, ask maintenance to try to reduce the background hum. Also, seek out quieter meeting spaces that have fewer acoustic distractions.

- Be aware of lighting. Rooms should be sufficiently well lit so that others can read your lips. Whether or not someone has an identified hearing loss, he or she might look at your face for extra clues about what you are saying. (Read more in "Environment of Care," starting on page 57.)

Think broadly about your Web site users. This includes not only those with vision loss but also Web users with cognitive or learning disabilities as well as those who seldom seek out digital information. There are many ways to make it easier for users to navigate your Web site and find the information they need. One of the best resources to learn more is the W3C Web Accessibility Initiative (www.w3.org/wai).

Design printed materials so they are easy to see and use. Consider the following elements in your design:

- *Contrast.* Sometimes one person's needs and preferences are the opposite of someone else's. For example, a person with low vision may prefer reverse contrast—light print on a dark background—while a person with normal vision may prefer dark lettering on a light background. Find ways to accommodate both preferences in the critical elements of your design. For example, you might use reverse contrast in key parts of a brochure (such as the title and headings) while using standard lettering in the body of the text. (Read more in "Know Your Audience: Vision Problems," starting on page 127.)
- *Font.* Choose a font that is not overly stylized and does not vary too much from what people are accustomed to seeing. People often have strong opinions about fonts. Some prefer serif fonts in which the letters have little "feet" or "wings." An example is Times New Roman, which is found in most word processing programs. Others favor sans serif fonts like Arial, which is a type of block lettering. And some favor type that looks like handwriting, such as Comic Sans. Many experts believe that the jury is still out as to which type of font works best. (Read more in "Document Design," starting on page 51.)
- *Type size.* For regular text, use a type size between 12 and 16 points. Type that is smaller than 12 points is hard for most people to see. Type that is larger than 16 points can result in more pages than most people want to read.
- *Line length.* People with low vision may have difficulty when there are too many words on a line; people with cognitive impairments may

have difficulty when there are too few. In general, most people prefer seven to 12 words in a line of continuous text. This relatively short line length can often be accomplished with columns (like in a newspaper), with two columns per page. Justify (line up evenly) the text on the left margin and keep the right margin ragged (uneven).

- *Pictures.* Choose pictures that have sufficient contrast between foreground and background. Crop the pictures so that they have a clear border around a central image.
- *Paper finish.* Glossy paper has a glare that can make it difficult for people with impaired vision to read. To increase legibility, use matte paper for all your printed materials.
- *User/experts.* User/experts represent the consumers or readers you are designing for. Solicit their opinion as you design written materials, asking about both appeal and usability.

Universal design describes a concept of designing products, environments, and communications that not only considers the specific needs of people with disabilities, but also takes into account the more universal changes that everyone faces as they age.

Citations

Osborne H (host). 2010, October 5. Universal Design and Health Communication [audio podcast]. *Health Literacy Out Loud,* no. 46. Available at http://healthliteracy .com/hlol-universal-design. Accessed February 18, 2011.

Osborne H. 2001, January. In Other Words . . . Communicating Across a Life Span . . . Universal Design in Print and Web-Based Communication. *On Call.* Available at http://www.healthliteracy.com/universal-design-in-communication. Accessed February 18, 2011.

Sources to Learn More

Bright K, Cook G. 2010. *The Colour, Light and Contrast Manual: Designing and Managing Inclusive Built Environments.* London: Wiley-Blackwell.

Institute for Human-Centered Design. Available at http://www.humancentereddesign .org/ and http://www.adaptenv.org/.

Keates SL, Clarkson PJ. 2003. *Countering Design Exclusion: An Introduction to Inclusive Design.* London: Springer-Verlag.

Norman DA. 2002. *The Design of Everyday Things.* New York: Basic Books.

Osborne H (host). 2009, December 7. Using Design to Get Readers to Read and Keep Reading [audio podcast]. *Health Literacy Out Loud,* no. 29. Available at http://www.healthliteracy.com/hlol-design-principles. Accessed February 18, 2011.

Preiser W, Smith KH (eds.). 2010. *Universal Design Handbook.* 2nd ed. Columbus, OH: McGraw-Hill Professional.

Schriver KA. 1996. *Dynamics in Document Design: Creating Texts for Readers.* New York: John Wiley & Sons.

Visuals

Visuals include artwork like pictographs (simple line drawings), photographs, anatomic diagrams, comics, and other images that convey actions or ideas. Many people enjoy and learn from visuals. This includes visual learners (those who learn best when seeing, reading, or being shown) as well as people with limited literacy or language skills who benefit from illustrations, not just words.

The airline industry is an example of doing this well, with picture-based emergency instructions provided at each seat. The same principles can be applied equally well to health materials, whether written as single-page fact sheets, fold-over brochures, or multi-page instructions.

Domenic Screnci, EdD, is the executive director of Educational Media and Technology at Boston University and also teaches Visual Literacy and Information Design at UMass Boston. In a *Health Literacy Out Loud* podcast, he spoke about visual literacy and health, saying that images can help people take in information faster and more accurately, and remember it better. Screnci talked of the importance of finding a "sweet spot" between words and visuals—balancing the use of both to reach the greatest audience, no matter their learning style (Osborne 2009, January 29).

Stories from Practice: Visuals Help Patients Understand

Here is a story a colleague shared with me. Herb, a 66-year-old general contractor, had a major heart attack several years ago. His doctor performed an emergency coronary angiography to examine the blood vessels and chambers of his heart. After the procedure, Herb's doctor explained what happened and gave him a simple line drawing of the heart and arteries. She colored in where each of his arteries was blocked and wrote alongside how much it was occluded.

Seeing so clearly what was wrong, Herb readily agreed to participate in a cardiac rehabilitation program and change his diet and exercise habits. In fact, Herb did so well that he was asked to speak with other patients who were just diagnosed with cardiovascular disease. To Herb's surprise and disappointment, not one of the more than 100 people he spoke with had ever been given a "heart picture" like his. They often comment how a drawing like the one Herb's doctor gave him could have helped them better understand their diagnosis and its treatment.

STRATEGIES, IDEAS, AND SUGGESTIONS

Here are some strategies to visually communicate health messages (Osborne 1999; 2008, May 8; 2008, August 21):

Acquire the artwork you need. There are many ways to acquire needed artwork. You might begin by looking online for free or low-cost visuals. I often start my search with Google Images at www.google.com/images. When you find an image you like, make sure you can freely use it or follow the instructions to obtain copyright permission. Another way is to ask a graphic artist, photographer, or cartoonist to create visuals specifically for you. I do this a lot and often work with Mark Tatro of Rotate Graphics (www.rotategraphics .com). And of course, there is always the option of creating your own artwork or asking an artistic colleague or friend to help.

Show sensitivity and respect. Choose visuals that not only are realistic but also show people at their best. For instance, when writing about general health issues, include some people who are active and not just ill or infirm.

As possible, represent the culture of your audience. This might include pictures of men wearing berets or turbans, not just baseball caps. And make sure that your artwork is as current as the text. This includes pictures with up-to-date hairstyles, clothing, and technology (such as cell phones and laptop computers).

Select visuals appropriate to the subject matter. For example, you might use humorous, cartoon-like characters when writing about well-baby care, but more subdued illustrations in booklets about serious diagnoses. Consider the color of paper, too. I still recall a fact sheet about colonoscopy instructions from many years ago. It was printed on light brown paper—not a good color choice, in my humble opinion.

Show people in their entirety, not just body parts. When writing about just one part of the body, such as the spleen, it's tempting to show only this aspect of the anatomy. Try, instead, to include at least one picture of the whole human body with the spleen clearly identified. This way, readers have a "road map" to see how large the spleen is and where it is located. Also, you avoid "disembodied body parts," which may be upsetting, especially to people traumatized by violence or war.

Combine pictures and text. Visuals alone are seldom sufficient, especially when explaining complicated information. To improve understanding, include simply worded captions beneath each visual. Captions not only help readers know what they're looking at but also reinforce key ideas and actions.

Appreciate that symbols are not always understood. Symbols, just like other types of visuals, are subject to interpretation. For example, a picture of a pill bottle alongside a knife and fork may be intended to show that medication should be taken with meals. But for those from countries where food is taken by hand from a common serving bowl, this symbol may not have meaning or relevance.

Consider the needs of those with visual or cognitive disabilities. Make visuals easy to see by having a lot of contrast. Generally, this means black ink on white, ivory, buff, or other light-colored or pastel paper. Don't rely solely on colorful print or drawings to convey your message. Some people cannot differentiate between two shades of the same color or may not be able to see colors at all. Also, avoid decorative backgrounds like watermarks and washes that make it hard for people to know where to focus attention. (Read more in "Document Design," starting on page 51.)

Confirm understanding. As with all forms of communication, make sure that your readers can understand and use visual information. For printed materials, ask your intended audience for their feedback, and confirm that your illustrations, colors, and symbols are appealing and informative. In person, you might confirm understanding by saying in a light-hearted way, "Let's see how good an artist I am. What does this picture mean to you?" (Read more in the "Confirm Understanding" chapters, starting on page 35.)

Stories from Practice: When You Are the Artist

Maybe you have an artistic flair or at least a willingness to draw pictures. Here is some advice when you are the artist:

- *Include the most important elements.* My dermatologist drew an impromptu picture of a mole she recently removed from my toe. She included only enough detail to show how far the mole had spread. This picture, even more than her words, reassured me that the diagnosis wasn't as dire as I feared.
- *Ask patients if they'd like to keep your drawing.* While you may think that your drawings are nothing special, patients may find them very helpful. Ask patients if they want to keep your drawing— even if you drew it on paper from the examining table (as the doctor did when sketching my mole). Then add a few key words so patients can accurately recall what your drawing means.
- *If you really lack artistic talent.* Consider using an illustrated sheet as a base and adding words, numbers, or highlighting to personalize the message. Naomi Karten wrote a humorous, but true, tale about "Dr. Scribbling," an orthopedist whose drawing wasn't on a par with his surgical prowess. You can find this story in the collection of Health Literacy Month stories at http://healthliteracy.com/hlmonth-scribbling. (Karten 2009, October).

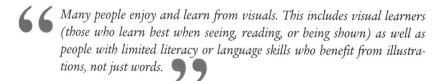

Many people enjoy and learn from visuals. This includes visual learners (those who learn best when seeing, reading, or being shown) as well as people with limited literacy or language skills who benefit from illustrations, not just words.

CITATIONS

Karten N. 2009, October. Knee News. *Health Literacy Month.* Available at http://healthliteracy.com/hlmonth-scribbling. Accessed July 17, 2010.

Osborne H. 1999. In Other Words . . . Teaching with Pictures. *On Call.* 2(11):38–39. Available at http://healthliteracy.com/teaching-with-pictures. Accessed July 15, 2010.

Osborne H. 2008, May 8. In Other Words . . . Using Visuals and Other Creative Tools to Make Health Messages Clear. *On Call.* Available at http://www.healthliteracy.com/visuals. Accessed July 15, 2010.

Osborne H. 2008, August 21. In Other Words . . . Using Comics to Communicate Your Health Message. *On Call.* Available at http://www.healthliteracy.com/comics. Accessed July 15, 2010.

Osborne H (host). 2009, January 29. Domenic Screnci Talks About Visual Literacy [audio podcast]. *Health Literacy Out Loud,* no. 9. Available at http://www.healthliteracy.com/hlol-visual-literacy. Accessed July 15, 2010.

SOURCES TO LEARN MORE

Carstens A, Maes A, Gangla-Birir L. 2006. Understanding Visuals in HIV/AIDS Education in South Africa: Differences Between Literate and Low-Literate Audiences. *African Journal of AIDS Research.* 5(3):221–232.

Delp C, Jones J. 1996. Communicating Information to Patients: The Use of Cartoon Illustrations to Improve Comprehension of Instructions. *Academic Emergency Medicine.* 3(3):264–270.

Doak CC, Doak LG, Root JH, 1996. Visuals and How to Use Them. Ch. 7 in *Teaching Patients with Low Literacy Skills.* 2nd ed. Available at http://www.hsph.harvard.edu/healthliteracy/resources/doak-book/index.html. Accessed February 19, 2011.

Hanks K, Belliston L, 1990. *Rapid Viz: A New Method for the Rapid Visualization of Ideas.* Menlo Park, CA: Crisp Publications.

Hill LH. 2008. The Role of Visuals in Communicating Health Information to Low Literate Adults. *Focus on Basics: Connecting Research and Practice.* 9(B):40–46. Available at http://www.ncsall.net/fileadmin/resources/fob/2008/fob_9b.pdf. Accessed July 15, 2010.

Houts PS, Bachrach R, Witmer JT, Tringali CA, Bucher JA, Localio RA. 1998. Using Pictographs to Enhance Recall of Spoken Medical Instructions. *Patient Education and Counseling.* 35(2):83–88.

Houts PS, Doak CC, Doak LG, Loscalzo MJ. 2006. The Role of Pictures in Improving Health Communication: A Review of Research on Attention, Comprehension, Recall, and Adherence. *Patient Education and Counseling.* 61(2):173–190.

Houts PS, Witmer JT, Egeth HE, Loscalzo MJ, Zabora JR. 2001. Using Pictographs to Enhance Recall of Spoken Medical Instructions II. *Patient Education and Counseling.* 43(3):231–242.

Katz MG, Kripalani S, Weiss BD. 2006. Use of Pictorial Aids in Medication Instructions: A Review of the Literature. *American Journal of Health-System Pharmacy.* 63:2391–2397.

Osborne H. 2006, March. Health Literacy: How Visuals Can Help Tell the Healthcare Story. *Journal of Visual Communication in Medicine*. 29(1):28–32. Available at http://www.healthliteracy.com/visuals-tell-health-literacy-story. Accessed April 6, 2011.

Osborne H (host). 2009, July 13. Developing Healthcare Materials With and For Village Health Workers [audio podcast]. *Health Literacy Out Loud*, no. 18. Available at http://www.healthliteracy.com/hlol-hesperian. Accessed February 20, 2011.

Rohret L, Ferguson KJ. 1990. Effective Use of Patient Education Illustrations. *Patient Education and Counseling*. 15(1):73–75.

Sonneman MR. 1997. *Beyond Words: A Guide to Drawing Out Ideas*. Berkeley, CA: Ten Speed Press.

Writing for the Web

STARTING POINTS

Many people look to Web sites for health information. "Web users" (people who go online for information) may look for help deciding whether they really need to see a doctor. If they find that they do, they might search online for names of local providers who offer a certain service. After appointments, Web users may search for additional information about tests and treatments the doctor recommended. And when Web users want additional support, they might participate in online chats and forums.

To learn about communicating clearly on the Web, I spoke with Janice (Ginny) Redish, PhD, who is an expert in plain language and Web writing and author of *Letting Go of the Words: Writing Web Content That Works*. In a *Health Literacy Out Loud* podcast, she said that people access information differently on the Web than they do in print. She compared the process of navigating Web sites to talking on the phone. Redish described it as a dynamic and interactive conversation, with Web users searching for a particular topic and then clicking links they think relevant or helpful. This contrasts to printed information, where readers follow the flow of information as organized by an author or editor (Osborne 2009, August 23).

Stories from Practice: Web Site for Users with Limited Literacy Skills

Healthfinder.gov is a Web site of the Office of Disease Prevention and Health Promotion (ODPHP) at the U.S. Department of Health and Human Services (HHS). It includes a tool designed for users with limited literacy skills called *Quick Guide to Healthy Living* (available at http://www.healthfinder.gov/prevention/). This is an easy-to-use and easy-to-read Web site with information on a wide range of disease prevention and wellness topics.

Stacy Robison, MPH, CHES, is a certified health educator and co-founder of the consulting company, CommunicateHealth. In a *Health Literacy Out Loud Podcast*, Robison talked about her experience writing and designing the *Quick Guide*. She spoke about the challenge of creating a site primarily for people with limited literacy or limited online experience. "A lot of people make the argument that people with limited literacy skills or limited experience on the Web aren't going online for health information," she says. But Robison considers this a self-fulfilling prophecy. "It's this puzzle that we can't get out of because we say there is no point in creating this Web content for people with limited literacy skills. At the same time, if we don't have any easy-to-understand or easy-to-use health information online, then folks with limited literacy skills aren't going to start using the Internet to search for health information."

Obviously, the *Quick Guide* is doing something right. It has been tested and developed with close to 800 Web users, most of who have limited health literacy skills. They say this Web site works well. I've tried it myself and wholeheartedly agree.

Source: Osborne (2010, March 23).

STRATEGIES, IDEAS, AND SUGGESTIONS

Here are some suggestions to consider (Osborne 2005, July; 2009, August 23; 2010, March 23):

Include standard conventions and pages that most visitors expect. These include:

- **Navigation bar.** Like a table of contents, the navigation bar is a clickable list of key topics and pages. It usually is located on the left or along the top of each Web page.

- **"About Us" page.** This is where users can check the source and credibility of information. It should include names and credentials of key people who created or sponsor the Web site.
- **"Contact Us" page.** For large organizations, this should include contact information for the sponsoring organization as well as its Web editor.
- **Headings.** Redish recommends using questions, statements, or verb phrases that connect people to specific information they are looking for. An example is a header such as "What is strep throat?"

Consider layout and design:

- Keep the most important messages in the middle and center of the screen. Based on user testing, Robison learned to keep key information centered and "above the fold" (at the top of the screen). This way, users do not need to scroll down or look on the left or right.
- Create small, stand-alone sections of text. This allows users to get a full piece of information without needing to scan and scroll through a whole page. During testing of the *Quick Guide to Healthy Living*, ODPHP found that users would skip over a paragraph when there were more than three lines of text. "That's not sentences, that's actual lines of text," said Robison.
- Make hypertext (links) evident with bright or contrasting colors. Red or blue are commonly used for these purposes. But also include alternatives such as symbols or text to make hyperlinks evident by users who are color blind or have limited vision.
- Use about half the number of words you might use in print. When lengthy materials cannot or should not be shortened, format information so users can easily print the pages rather than reading onscreen.

Make the site accessible. This means considering the needs of people with disabilities as well as of those with older computers or slower connections. Here are some ways:

- Use simple photographs, illustrations, diagrams, or other graphics. More complex designs can take a long time to download or slow down the process of going from page to page.
- Consider whether to have a text-only version. For years, it was recommended to have just text and not also graphics or other visual features. This would help those with slower computers and also people who use screen readers to read text aloud. But Redish says that this

recommendation is changing. One reason is that text-only versions are often not maintained and updated as much as the "real" site. Redish says another reason is that "Blind and low-vision users in our usability studies disdained text-only versions. They wanted the 'real' site to be accessible." (Redish 2011).

- "Test-drive" your Web site on a slower or older machine. You might be able to do this is by going online at a public computer (such as at a library or senior center) to see how well your Web site works.
- Learn more about making Web sites accessible. An excellent Web site to explore is W3C, the Web Accessibility Initiative (http://www .w3.org/WAI/).

Test with your intended audience. Can Web users understand and make use of your information? Can they easily navigate from one section to another? The answers to these as well as many other questions can be learned through usability testing. This means watching people who represent your audience as they try out your Web site.

Robison said that user testing with people who have limited literacy skills was key when designing the *Quick Guide* Web site. "If they don't find what they're looking for or they're not able to do the task, as the Web designer and the Web writer, you go back and fix it. It's never a fault of the user." Robison adds, "If people don't understand and they're not finding the information, then we need to go back to the drawing board and do our jobs better" (Osborne 2010, March 23). (Read more in "Confirming Understanding: Feedback," starting on page 35.)

Can Web users understand and make use of your information? Can they easily navigate from one section to another? The answers to these as well as many other questions can be learned through usability testing.

CITATIONS

Osborne H. 2005, July. In Other Words . . . What Makes Web Sites Patient-Friendly? *On Call.* Available at http://healthliteracy.com/patient-friendly-websites. Accessed August 24, 2010.

Osborne H (host). 2009, August 23. Communicating Clearly on the Web [audio podcast]. *Health Literacy Out Loud,* no. 19. Available at http://healthliteracy .com/hlol-web. Accessed February 19, 2011.

Osborne H (host). 2010, March 23. Creating Usable, Useful Health Websites for Readers at All Levels [audio podcast]. *Health Literacy Out Loud,* no. 34. Available at http://healthliteracy.com/hlol-websites-for-all-readers. Accessed August 23, 2010.

Redish J. 2011. Personal communication.

SOURCES TO LEARN MORE

Eichner J, Dullabh P. 2007, October. *Accessible Health Information Technology (Health IT) for Populations with Limited Literacy: A Guide for Developers and Purchasers of Health IT.* Prepared for the National Opinion Research Center for Health IT. AHRQ publication no 08-0010-EF. Rockville, MD: Agency for Healthcare Research and Quality.

Fox S. 2008, August 26. *The Engaged e-Patient Population.* Pew Internet & American Life Project. Available at http://www.pewinternet.org/~/media//Files/Reports/2008/PIP_Health_Aug08.pdf.pdf. Accessed August 5, 2010.

Gualtieri LN. 2009. *The Doctor as the Second Opinion and the Internet as the First.* CHI 2009, April 4–9, 2009. Available at http://lisaneal.files.wordpress.com/2009/02/alt12-gualtieri1.pdf. Accessed August 23, 2010.

Hackos JAT, Redish JC. 1997. *User and Task Analysis for Interface Design.* New York: John Wiley & Sons.

Jensen JD, King AJ, Davis LA, Guntzviller LM. 2010. Utilization of Internet Technology by Low-Income Adults: The Role of Health Literacy, Health Numeracy, and Computer Assistance. *Journal of Aging and Health.* 22(6):804–826.

National Institute on Aging and the National Library of Medicine. 2001. *Making Your Web Site Senior Friendly: A Checklist.* Washington, DC: Author. Available at www.nih.gov/icd/od/ocpl/resources/wag/documents/checklist.pdf. Accessed August 24, 2010.

The Plain Language Action and Information Network (PLAIN). Available at http://www.plainlanguage.gov/.

Redish J. 2007. *Letting Go of the Words: Writing Web Content That Works.* Boston: Elsevier/Morgan Kaufmann.

Rubin J, Chisnell D. 2008. *Handbook of Usability Testing: How to Plan, Design, and Conduct Effective Tests.* 2nd ed. Indianapolis, IN: Wiley.

Taylor H (ed.). 2008. Number of "Cyberchondriacs"—Adults Going Online for Health Information—Has Plateaued or Declined. *Harris Interactive Healthcare News.* 8(8):1–6.

Yellowlees P. 2009, April 2. The Internet—A Third "Person" in Our Consulting Rooms. *Medscape Business of Medicine.* Available at http://www.medscape.com/viewarticle/589642. Accessed August 5, 2010.

Usability.gov. U.S. Department of Health and Human Services. Available at http://usability.gov/.

U.S. Department of Health and Human Services, Centers for Medicare and Medicaid Services. 2010. *Toolkit for Making Written Material Clear and Effective.* Available at http://www.cms.gov/WrittenMaterialsToolkit/. Accessed January 12, 2011.

U.S. Department of Health and Human Services, Office of Disease Prevention and Health Promotion. 2009, October 19. *Health Literacy Online: Building an Easy-to-Use Health Information Web Site.* Available at http://healthliteracy.com/hlmonth-building-website. Accessed February 19, 2011.

U.S. Department of Health and Human Services, Office of Disease Prevention and Health Promotion. 2010. *Health Literacy Online: A Guide to Writing and Designing Easy-to-Use Health Web Sites,* Washington, DC: Author. Available at http://www.health.gov/healthliteracyonline/. Accessed April 6, 2011.

Useit.com. Jakob Nielsen's Web site about usable information technology. Available at http://www.useit.com/.

X-tras

STARTING POINTS

X-tras (or "extras" for spelling enthusiasts) make programs unique and yours. Always creative and often fun, extras include "far-out" ideas, "out-of-the-box" thinking, and "off-the-wall" communication strategies that can help people better understand health information.

Extras aren't just entertaining. Indeed, they are rooted in the philosophy that people have more capacity to learn when they are relaxed and having fun. Additionally, most extras are multimodal and appeal to people's varied learning styles of seeing, doing, listening, and interacting. Extras are effective with audiences of all ages and abilities, including health professionals, patients, students, and the general public.

Creativity drives many of these extras. Whether inspired and developed by just one person, a whole department, or the entire organization, creative extras can provide education and information to meet today's healthcare challenges. Even one person can make a creative difference. What's needed is passion for an idea, willingness to take a risk, and commitment to follow through.

STRATEGIES, IDEAS, AND SUGGESTIONS

Here are some x-tra suggestions to use in practice (Law 2010; Osborne 2008, March 20; 2008, October 2; 2010, February 23):

Get creative. Admittedly, some people are naturally more creative than others. But even those who believe they are not creative can learn to think in more innovative ways. When I supervised occupational therapy students, for example, we often faced clinical situations in which traditional interventions didn't work or didn't work well. To help the students come up with alternative treatment solutions, I asked them to participate in two creativity exercises, "making the strange familiar" and "making the familiar strange." These exercises helped the students think of old problems in new ways so that they could then apply creative thinking to clinical challenges.

Stories from Practice: Using Puppets to Teach About Health

The St. Louis Christian Chinese Community Service Center in St. Louis, Missouri, uses puppetry to teach its members about ways to talk with health care providers. For many within the Chinese community, especially elders, speaking up to doctors and asking a lot of questions is new and often difficult to do.

Harold Law, DSc, Vice Chair of the Board of Directors for the Chinese Community Center, explains that puppets have conveyed important messages for thousands of years in China. He thought that puppetry could be an effective way to convey health literacy concepts, too.

Law, along with others, created a 10-minute puppet show about health communication. The show includes five characters (doctor, patient, family member, nurse, and interpreter) who essentially role-play a scenario of effective health communication. The goal is to encourage community members to speak up and ask questions. Puppetry seems to work well. In an audience discussion immediately after the puppet show, an older woman shared, "I never knew I could ask the doctor so many questions."

Law sees puppetry as a nonintrusive, nonthreatening way to communicate memorable health messages. He says that puppetry can be adapted for audiences of all ages, cultures, and languages. He envisions exciting possibilities ahead, such as a puppet show about smoking cessation. His biggest hurdle, however, is technical—finding a puppet that smokes! (To see the puppet show, go to http://www.vimeo.com/12828087).

Source: Health Literacy Missouri (2010); Law (2010).

Know your audience. Whether your innovative idea is geared more for students, patients, health professionals, or the general public, learn about your intended audience. Know about their literacy, language, culture, and learning needs. Be sensitive, as well, to people's capacity for humor, tolerance for uncertainty, and willingness to try something innovative, fun, and new.

Make it easy for others to support your innovative project. X-tra ideas are seldom in the budget. Almost always, it takes another dose of creativity to get needed staff, funding, and other resources. Let internal funders know how this project can help generate income (such as by enrolling new patients) or reduce expenses (like decreasing re-hospitalizations). Consider partnering with like-minded groups or asking local foundations for grants to help sponsor your project.

Here are some examples of X-tras:

- *Contests.* Several years ago I wanted to come up with a tagline for the Health Literacy Month logo. Given that this initiative has a budget of zero outside dollars, I created a "tagline contest." The prize was 100 Health Literacy Month postcards and unlimited bragging rights. Results were amazing, with more than 50 submissions from health professionals as well as advertising agencies. Thanks to this contest, Kenneth Lo, then at the New York City Department of Health and Mental Hygiene, came up with the terrific tagline, "Finding the right words for better health."
- *Celebrity news.* Michelle Berman, MD, brings not only experience as a pediatrician but also an interest in using celebrity news to teach about health. She and her physician-husband wanted to make the most of "teachable moments," situations in which people are receptive to information that can lead to healthy behaviors. And so they created the Celebrity Diagnosis Web site (http://celebritydiagnosis.com), which features health news about athletes, politicians, and movie stars. It even has a story about Santa Claus getting a flu shot because he was concerned about getting sick from children sitting on his lap. "If you give people information in fun and different ways, they'll take it," says Berman (Osborne 2010, February 23).
- *Music and song.* Mache Seibel, MD, is an advocate of using music and song to teach positive health messages. Seibel writes, produces, and performs songs about health and wellness for people of all ages. He says that music can communicate important information in a format that people can retain and act on. "If you can sing about, you can talk about. If you can talk about it, you can take action. And once something becomes actionable, you can change it," Seibel says (Osborne 2008, March 20; 2008, October 2).

Whether inspired and developed by just one person, a whole department, or the entire organization, creative extras can provide education and information to meet today's healthcare challenges. What's needed is passion for an idea, willingness to take a risk, and commitment to follow through. **99**

CITATIONS

Health Literacy Missouri. 2010. *Chinese Puppets—St. Louis Christian Chinese Community Service Center* [video]. Available at http://www.vimeo.com/12828087. Accessed February 14, 2011.

Law H. 2010. Phone interview.

Osborne H. 2008, March 20. In Other Words . . . Using Music and Song as Tools of Health Communication. *On Call.* Available at http://www.healthliteracy.com/music-song. Accessed August 23, 2010.

Osborne H (host). 2008, October 2. Mache Seibel Talks about Using Music and Song [audio podcast]. *Health Literacy Out Loud,* no. 2. Available at http://www.healthliteracy.com/hlol-music-song. Accessed August 23, 2010.

Osborne H (host). 2010, February 23. Teachable Moments: Using Celebrity to Teach About Health [audio podcast]. *Health Literacy Out Loud,* no. 32. Available at http://www.healthliteracy.com/hlol-celebrity. Accessed August 23, 2010.

SOURCES TO LEARN MORE

Cueva M, Kuhnley R, Lanier A, Dignan M. 2005. Using Theater to Promote Cancer Education in Alaska. *Journal of Cancer Education.* 20(1):45–48.

Daitz B. 2011, January 24. With Poem, Broaching the Topic of Death. *New York Times.* Available at http://www.nytimes.com/2011/01/25/health/25navajo.html. Accessed February 14, 2011.

HealthRock. Available at http://www.healthrock.com.

Huron D. 2008. Science and Music: Lost in Music. *Nature.* 453(7194):456–457.

Lawson PJ, Flocke SA. 2009. Teachable Moments for Health Behavior Change: A Concept Analysis. *Patient Education and Counseling.* 76(1):25–30.

Mache Seibel, MD. http://www.mseibelmd.com/.

Osborne H (host). 2009, October 14. Teaching and Singing about Health in South Africa [audio podcast]. *Health Literacy Out Loud,* no. 25. Available at http://www.healthliteracy.com/hlol-south-africa-songs. Accessed August 23, 2010.

Peterson DA, Thaut MH. 2007. Music Increases Frontal EEG Coherence During Verbal Learning. *Neuroscience Letters.* 412(3):217–221.

Seibel MM. 2006. Health Through Music and Song. *Sexuality, Reproduction and Menopause.* 4(2):46–47.

You: Empathy and Humanity

STARTING POINTS

In addition to knowledge, skills, and experience, you bring "you" to each patient encounter. "You" includes empathy—sensitivity to another person's feelings, thoughts, and experiences. "You" also includes humanity—responding to patients in caring ways that you would want for yourself.

Empathy and humanity go a long way to improve health communication. When patients feel valued and listened to, they likely will relax and be more receptive to learning new health information, even when that news is scary or sad. But when patients feel they are being treated in an impersonal or judgmental manner, they may well "tune out" and not fully process what providers are telling them or asking that they do.

STRATEGIES, IDEAS, AND SUGGESTIONS

Here are some ideas to consider (Crannell 2004; Osborne 2005, May/June; 2005, October; 2007, May; 2008, November 13):

Develop rapport. Set a tone for good communication by developing rapport with each patient. In office appointments, you can begin by briefly chatting about nonmedical matters and then asking patients what they want to focus on today. When talking about diagnoses and treatment options, find out how much information patients want to know and to what extent they are willing to participate in decision making. (Read more in "Decision Aids & Shared Decision-Making," starting on page 45.)

Stories from Practice: A Father's Story of Unfortunate Communication

---

Here is a story a friend shared about his family's experience. Ken's son Chuck has many moles. When Chuck was 12 years old, his doctor biopsied two of his moles in a rather unpleasant procedure. A few days later on a stormy New Year's Eve afternoon, the doctor called from a pay phone to tell Ken about the test results. "I just received a report that your son has melanoma. We need to remove it right away."

Not expecting the call that day and startled by the bad news, Ken's first thought was of the unpleasant biopsy. When Ken asked, "What happens if you don't remove it?" he expected to hear about treatment alternatives. Ken was dumbfounded when the doctor said, "Then your son has only eight months to live."

More than 20 years later, Ken still vividly remembers this call. While thankful that Chuck's melanoma was successfully removed (by another doctor), Ken remains upset about what he feels was an insensitive, thoughtless manner in which this physician communicated bad news.

Make sure that now is a good time to talk. Empathy is conveyed as much by actions and timing, as with words. Use eye contact, body posture, and tone of voice to let patients know they have your full attention. As well, make sure patients are fully focused on what you are saying. Make it clear what needs to be discussed right now or could wait until a more convenient time.

In the story above, it is easy to see how ill timed the phone call was between Ken and the doctor. The doctor was obviously rushed and even commented that he was calling from a pay phone in a rainy parking lot. Likewise, Ken was distracted by a having houseful of guests for New Year's Eve. Talking at another time would have benefitted them both.

Take cues about pacing from the patient. Doing so can help you determine how quickly, or slowly, to present information. In Ken's case, the doctor rapidly jumped to the grimmest news possible. In replaying this conversation, Ken says he would have preferred it if the doctor had slowed down and first eased his concerns about the needed excision. Only if and when Ken raised the issue of long-term prognosis should the doctor have addressed it.

Decide whether to share personal experiences. Some patients are comforted when their providers share a personal experience, such as being in a situation similar to the patient's. Before disclosing personal information, however, make sure the patient and family are receptive to you doing so. While some might find your openness helpful and supportive, others may feel that your experience is too much for them to deal with now. As well, consider your motives and make sure that you are revealing personal information solely for the patient's benefit, not yours. (Read more in "Know Your Audience: Emotion," starting on page 105.)

Offer Hope. Almost universally, patients want hope. Even when dealing with progressive illnesses, patients and families appreciate it when their providers offer encouragement and support their goals. Says Ken of a much more empathetic provider, "She didn't give up hope for us. We respond to hope."

 Empathy and humanity go a long way to improve health communication. When patients feel valued and listened to, they likely will relax and be more receptive to learning new health information, even when that news is scary or sad.

Citations

Crannell K. 2004. Personal communication.

Osborne H. 2005, May/June. In Other Words . . . Communicating Bad and Sad News. *On Call*. Available at http://www.healthliteracy.com/bad-sad-news. Accessed February 19, 2011.

Osborne H. 2005, October. In Other Words . . . Know When to Speak and When to Listen . . . Communicating with People Who Are Anxious or Angry. *On Call*. Available at http://www.healthliteracy.com/anxious-angry-patients. Accessed April 5, 2011.

Osborne H. 2007, May. In Other Words . . . When Patients and Providers Talk About Health. *On Call*. Available at http://www.healthliteracy.com/patients-providers. Accessed February 19, 2011.

Osborne H. 2008, November 13. In Other Words . . . Talking with Patients About Touchy Subjects. *On Call*. Available at http://www.healthliteracy.com/touchy-subjects. Accessed February 19, 2011.

Sources to Learn More

Osborne H. 2006, May/June. In Other Words . . . Communicating When Naked: My Perspective as a Patient. *On Call*. Available at http://www.healthliteracy.com/communicating-when-naked. Accessed February 19, 2011.

Osborne H (host). 2011, June 28. The Importance of Empathy in Health Communication. *Health Literacy Out Loud*, no. 61. Available at http://healthliteracy.com/hlol-empathy. Accessed July 5, 2011.

The Schwartz Center for Compassionate Healthcare. Available at http://www.theschwartzcenter.org/. Includes information on Schwartz Center Rounds®.

Zest and Pizzazz

STARTING POINTS

Zest and pizzazz include the commitment and passion that you bring to health literacy. These qualities are also about the energy that sustains and motivates you to continue. Admittedly, it's fairly easy to remain enthused when colleagues rave about your new health literacy workshop or when patients beam with understanding after you draw pictures to explain their diagnosis.

But it can be much harder to maintain the momentum when you must explain, yet again, what health literacy is and why it matters. Or when you have colleagues who still don't "get it" and continue communicating in ways that are neither effective nor understandable. And it can indeed be exhausting to continually search for funding needed to sustain health literacy programs that you know are worthwhile.

Through good times and bad, it helps a lot to remember why you care so much about health literacy. Whether your motivation is personal, or professional, or a bit of both, keep in mind that health literacy is everyone's responsibility. As a dear friend and colleague once said to me, "If you don't keep advocating for health literacy, who will?"

Stories from Practice: Why Health Literacy Matters

I founded Health Literacy Month (www.healthliteracymonth.org) in 1999 as a way to raise awareness about the need for understandable health information. I envisioned this as a time when health literacy advocates would speak with a collective voice—together letting the whole world know about the importance of clear, simple, and understandable health communication.

For 10 years, organizations had been hosting their own Health Literacy Month events. In 2009, I added something new. Inspired by Jay Allison, who produced the NPR radio show *This I Believe,* I created our own collection of stories, titled "Why Health Literacy Matters: Sharing Our Stories in Words, Pictures, and Sounds."

A terrific team of volunteers and I worked hard to gather, edit, and post a wide range of personal stories about why health literacy matters. The stories were told by patients, parents, caregivers, adult learners, graduate students, professors, clinicians, Web developers, librarians, public health specialists, and health educators from the United States, Canada, the United Kingdom, and Africa.

Individually and collectively, these stories make a poignant and powerful case why health literacy matters. Their zest and pizzazz remind us why we feel so passionate about this work. You can read, listen to, and watch all these stories by going to the Health Literacy Month Web site at www.healthliteracymonth.org.

STRATEGIES, IDEAS, AND SUGGESTIONS

Here are some ways to add health literacy zest and pizzazz (Osborne 2009):

Find your passion. Health literacy is seldom in anyone's job description. To have the energy to keep going, remember why health literacy matters. You may recall a personal experience as a patient or family member when health communication worked exceptionally well, or particularly badly. You may remember a patient who stared blankly when you gave her a brochure and another who grinned with understanding when you drew him a picture. Zest and pizzazz start with understanding why you are so passionate about health literacy.

Take risks. Health literacy is a fairly new concept. Figuring out how you can make a difference may, at times, feel like going on a journey without a map. For some, it is exciting to forge a path that others can later follow. For others, it is uncomfortable venturing into the unknown.

If you, like me, are willing to take some risks, then health literacy includes trying the untested. Sometimes what we do will work well, sometimes it won't. Regardless of the outcome, we almost certainly will learn something new. And to me, that's the key to navigating this health literacy journey.

Develop a support network. It's hard to remain enthused when you feel like you are the only health literacy advocate around. I know from experience that it helps to be part of a network that shares common goals. (Read more in "Organizational Efforts," starting on page 151.)

Some networks meet in person, bringing together organizations with common challenges and goals. Networks might include people from health care facilities, literacy programs, libraries, social service agencies, and the public at large. Online networks can be helpful, too. I learn a tremendous amount from the hundreds of health and literacy colleagues who participate in the LINCS Health Literacy Discussion List—an online discussion group sponsored by the Literacy Information and Communication System at http://lincs.ed.gov/mailman/listinfo/ Healthliteracy/.

Learn from those around you. Health literacy is bigger than any one person, profession, or program. A lot of my knowledge comes from others who share similar, yet not identical, communication challenges. For example, I learned so much from my neighbor, who teaches middle school students who come from foreign lands and speak other languages. I appreciate the power of drawing when artists convey complex ideas with just a few lines and squiggles. I value the simplicity of words when reading succinct, yet eloquent, essays. And when patients and family members tell me how hard it is to understand health information, I again remember why I do this work. Look around. The world is filled with health literacy zest and pizzazz.

 Health literacy is everyone's responsibility. As a dear friend and colleague once said to me, "If you don't keep advocating for health literacy, who will?"

CITATIONS

Osborne H. 2009. *Health Literacy Month Handbook: The Event Planning Guide for Health Literacy Advocates.* Available at http://healthliteracy.com/hlmonth-handbook. Accessed August 25, 2010.

SOURCES TO LEARN MORE

Osborne H (host). 2009, February 9. Julie McKinney Talks About an Online Health Literacy Community [audio podcast]. *Health Literacy Out Loud,* no. 10. Available at http://healthliteracy.com/hlol-online-community. Accessed February 19, 2011.

Osborne H (host). 2009, March 23. Len and Ceci Doak Discuss Health Literacy's Past, Present, and Future [audio podcast]. *Health Literacy Out Loud,* no. 13. Available at http://healthliteracy.com/hlol-doaks. Accessed February 19, 2011.

Osborne H (host). 2009, May 4. Dr. Rima Rudd Talks About the Health Literacy Burden in Healthcare [audio podcast]. *Health Literacy Out Loud,* no. 15. Available at http://healthliteracy.com/hlol-rima-rudd. Accessed February 19, 2011.

Osborne H (host). 2009, June 23. Dr. Arthur Culbert Talks About Statewide Health Literacy Initiatives [audio podcast]. *Health Literacy Out Loud,* no. 17. Available at http://healthliteracy.com/hlol-statewide-initiatives. Accessed February 19, 2011.

Osborne H (host). 2010, June 8. National Action Plan to Improve Health Literacy. *Health Literacy Out Loud,* no. 39. Available at http://healthliteracy.com/hlol-national-health-literacy-action-plan. Accessed August 25, 2010.

Osborne H. 2011. *Checklists for Health Literacy Month Events.* Available at http://healthliteracy.com/hlmonth-checklists. Accessed July 12, 2011.

U.S. Department of Health and Human Services, Office of Disease Prevention and Health Promotion. 2010. *National Action Plan to Improve Health Literacy.* Available at http://www.health.gov/communication/HLActionPlan. Accessed April 5, 2011.

Checklist:
Using This Book
in Practice

Health Literacy from A to Z: Practical Ways to Communicate Your Health Message, Second Edition is filled with hundreds of practical how-to strategies to meet health communication challenges. Being in practice, you may be using many of these strategies now. Other strategies may be new. Or perhaps there are ones you haven't used in a while.

This checklist is intended as a tool to remind and encourage you to put these strategies into day-to-day practice. It can also be a useful tool to inspire colleagues to take action. Imagine how understandable health care would be if everyone in practice used all these communication strategies, all the time.

☐ **Know your audience.** Effective health communication often takes more than a "one size fits all" approach. Know about those you are trying to reach with your health message. Have a sense of their learning needs (should you teach with pictures, use everyday words?), goals (what does your audience want or need to learn?), and interests (why does this topic matter to them, now?).

☐ **Work as a team.** Health literacy is about mutual understanding. It does not happen by one person communicating alone. Make a commitment to learn from, partner with, and otherwise work as a team with those on the receiving end of your health communication. Teamwork is needed at all stages—from developing messages, creating materials, and building programs, to measuring the success of all your communication efforts.

❑ **Create an environment of mutual understanding.** This is much more than a comfortable, private space. Communicate in a manner and tone that allow others to comfortably think, disagree, and ask questions. Yes, this may take some extra time at first. But consider the long-term benefit when those you are communicating with can truly understand and act on your health message.

❑ **Communicate in whatever ways work.** People learn and communicate in a variety of ways. Beyond just talking or using written materials, consider options like metaphors, pictures, puppets, music, and models. You do not need to choose just one. Often, it's more effective to communicate in multiple and creative ways.

❑ **Measure success.** What do you hope to accomplish with your health message? Specifically, what do you want the other person to know, do, and feel as a result? Identify these goals at the start of all communication projects. And then use these goals as a tool to identify problems and measure success.

❑ **Confirm understanding.** Communication is effective only when the other person understands. Confirm what people do and do not know. When there are gaps, rephrase; do not just repeat information. Make sure, as well, that you truly understand what the other person is communicating to you.

Checklist:
Using This Book
to Teach

Health literacy is a "hot topic" in classrooms and training programs today. Whether you are teaching health literacy as a semester-long course, giving a one-time lecture, or encouraging students to focus on health literacy as independent study, here is a checklist about ways to teach with *Health Literacy from A to Z.*

When you want students to know health literacy:

❏ A good chapter to start with is "About Health Literacy." This provides an overall introduction to the topic. Then follow the links and resources to find up-to-date research and data. Students may be more receptive to learning about health literacy once they see it's a problem that merits attention.

❏ To teach why each topic is important, focus on the introductory information at the beginning of each chapter. I refer to this section as "Starting Points." The information provides context for each issue and strategy that follows.

❏ For assignments, you might ask students to report on one or more of the references listed at the end of each chapter. Beyond exploring these articles, books, Web sites, and podcasts, encourage students to add their opinions about why this topic matters and ways they might help improve health understanding.

❑ Localize health literacy by having students survey others about a particular topic or strategy. They could do this with a short poll, brief questionnaire, or one-to-one conversation with patients, community members, or family.

When you want students to feel that health literacy matters:

❑ Students need to feel that learning is relevant to their goals. Help students appreciate why health literacy matters by asking them to read and reflect on the first-person accounts found in each chapter. I refer to these as "Stories from Practice."

❑ Ask students to write their own stories—focusing on their own experiences when health communication went wonderfully well, or horribly wrong. Health literacy matters when students feel that issues are personal and real.

When you want students to take action:

❑ Ask students to choose one or two items listed in "Strategies, Ideas, and Suggestions." Then have them try this through role-play with peers, practice on family and friends, or observation in clinical settings.

❑ After students gain experience and confidence with a strategy, ask them to teach it to others. If each student teaches a different strategy, at the end of a semester your class will have familiarity with a wide range of topics.

❑ Make it easy for students to take action. Ask them to commit to doing one of these strategies each day for the next two weeks. This way, you not only reinforce lessons learned but also encourage good communication habits.

Checklist:
Using This Book
with Patients

Health Literacy from A to Z is written especially for health professionals. Throughout, you will find ideas to share with patients. Here is a checklist of actions you might suggest patients do. Or do these actions yourself, when you are the patient.

- ☐ **Ask questions.** Even though it may feel awkward or rude, ask questions and let your doctor or other healthcare provider know if you do not understand something he or she has said. Sometimes it is hard to think of what to ask. You can start building a good question list by going to the Questions Are the Answer Web site from the federal Agency for Healthcare Research and Quality at http://www.ahrq.gov/questionsaretheanswer/.

- ☐ **Describe symptoms.** Be specific. Talk about when your symptoms started and how long they last. Use numbers and words to describe pain. Numbers can be from 1 to 10, with 10 being the worst pain you have ever had. You can also use words such as "achy," "tingly," or "sharp."

- ☐ **Keep track of your health history.** Be ready to answer questions about your health history, including any illnesses, medicines, and allergies. One way to keep track of this history is by making a notebook with places to write about:

  - Present illness, chronic conditions, and other health problems
  - Prescription medicines, over-the-counter drugs, and herbal remedies

- Instructions, including discharge forms as well as procedure preparations
- Immunizations and other shots
- Tests and test results
- Insurance information and healthcare proxy
- Names and phone numbers of close family members or friends
- Questions you want to ask, along with space to write the answers

❑ **Ask someone to go to appointments with you.** It can be hard to speak up—especially when you are feeling scared, sick, or in pain. Ask someone you know and trust (such as a family member or friend) to go to appointments with you. He or she can help by listening, remembering, taking notes, and asking questions.

❑ **Tell the healthcare provider if you have trouble hearing, seeing, reading, or understanding English.**

- If you wear a hearing aid or use eyeglasses, make sure to take these with you to all medical appointments.
- Tell the healthcare provider if he or she is speaking too softly or if the print on a brochure is too small to read.
- Make sure you understand. Repeat back, in your own words, what the healthcare provider said. Or demonstrate actions you plan to take. You might start by saying something like, "I want to make sure I understand this correctly. When you said to ____, that means I should ___. Is that correct?"

Index